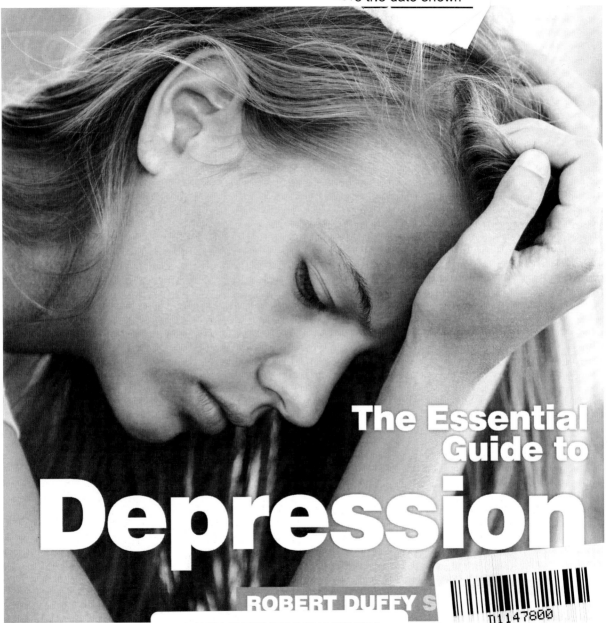

The Essential Guide to
Depression

ROBERT DUFFY

Published in Great Britain in 2019 by
need2know
Remus House
Coltsfoot Drive
Peterborough
PE2 9BF
Telephone 01733 898103
www.need2knowbooks.co.uk

Contents

Chapter 7: Health Problems Connected to Depression 67

Chapter 8: Looking Forward: Life with Depression 79

Help List 88

Sources 101

Introduction

I n our everyday lives, we tend to use the word "depressed" quite a lot. Certain colours are "depressing" and films about certain themes are "depressing". If we don't get the car loan we applied for or the promotion we were hoping for, we feel depressed. If we have a fight with a friend or loved one, or even just walk to the shop before realising we've forgotten our wallets, we're depressed.

Most of us get over the blue feeling in a matter of hours or less and soon we're involved in some other activity and the dark mood is forgotten. Real depression is quite different from these everyday uses of the word. The World Health Organisation estimates that approximately 450 million people worldwide experience mental health problems, with depression the predominant diagnosis. Statistics show anxiety and depression to be the most common combination of mental health disorders in the UK.

For the very depressed, even managing to get up and take care of personal hygiene is a major triumph, one which may seem beyond their ability as depression robs them of not only the energy but the desire to deal with their everyday activities. Someone experiencing clinical depression may describe it as feeling like all the colour has been drained from the world – it alters every aspect of life.

According to a study by the World Health Organisation, Global Burden of Disease and Risk Factors (2006) depression is the leading cause of disability for people aged 15 and older. It can be a steady drain on their inner resources and result in the loss of friends, job, career and lifestyle. Things that once interested or delighted them suddenly seem pointless; getting out of bed or leaving the house can seem like an unachievable goal, and life doesn't seem worth the effort any longer.

A depressed person may even attempt suicide if their depression is very severe, as they may find life not worth living.

A low mood can drag on for weeks, months or even years for a person with clinical depression. In some cases, clinical depression can even prove fatal.

You are not alone if you are experiencing depression. You might be surprised to learn that depression is an equal opportunity ailment. In the USA it is estimated that each year 12% of women, 7% of men and 4% of adolescents experience depression – about 23% of the population. At any one time, according to some estimates, approximately one in 10 men and one in four women in Britain are suffering from depression.

Between 2-6% of children and adolescents in the UK have depression, according to a report by the Royal College of General Practitioners. Worryingly, this report also suggested that the majority of depressive episodes in this age group will last between seven and nine months, with almost 50% experiencing a second episode within two years and up to 66% having another within five years.

Of all the disabling illnesses recognised in the world, the World Health Organisation lists depression within its top ten. The problem may be even bigger than we know, though, as it's difficult to get an accurate international picture. In certain countries, mental health problems carry such a stigma that people are reluctant to seek treatment.

The revered American president Abraham Lincoln suffered from 'melancholia', what we now call depression. Winston Churchill, whom some call the greatest ever British political leader, referred to his depression as 'a black dog' overshadowing his life. Depression has been an issue for many well-known people, from political and business leaders to popular celebrities.

Even Buzz Aldrin, the celebrated American astronaut, admits to having experienced depression, as has footballer Terry Bradshaw. In the acting area, well-known stars such as Hugh Laurie, Brooke Shields, Emma Thompson, Drew Carey, Harrison Ford… the list of stars who battle depression is a long one. It's believed that an episode of schizophrenia or manic depression (more commonly referred to as bipolar disorder) was what prompted the famous artist Vincent Van Gogh to have cut his ear off.

Depression has also been publicly discussed by contemporary writers like Anne Rice and Amy Tan. Rice believes that her depression stems from a long term illness and grief following the death of her husband, while Tan has explained that depression is an issue for her family as a whole.

Depression is known to have had an effect on the lives of many people in the music industry, including Brian Wilson of the Beach Boys, Nick Drake, Sheryl Crow, Trent Reznor of Nine-Inch Nails and Kurt Cobain. You could say you're in illustrious company if you've been diagnosed with depression!

A key to coping is to understand what is involved, to recognise warning signs, and to know when to seek help and what kind of help you need. No two cases of depression are the same, as the illness comes in several different types and severities. You can begin to take back control of your life and your condition if you arm yourself with all the knowledge you need and an understanding of where and when to get help.

Disclaimer

This book is not intended to replace medical advice although it can be used alongside it. The author of this book advises that he does not have medical qualifications, and that this book is intended only as a source of general information about depression. It is vital that you seek medical advice from a healthcare professional, such as your GP, if you are depressed or suspect you may have depression.

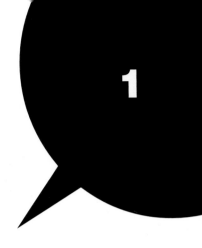

1

The Many Faces
of Depression

Depression can last for days, weeks, or even years. Each person experiences depression differently, but the symptoms range from constantly feeling tired, having no appetite, or eating too much; being unable to sleep or unable to get up in the morning; all the way through to thoughts or attempts at suicide. It becomes a 'Catch 22' situation where the depressed person's sense of worthlessness is reinforced as friends stop coming around, promotions go to someone else, exams are failed, dreams fall by the wayside and loved ones gradually lose patience.

There is no point in telling someone who is depressed to 'get over it' or to 'stop being so miserable, count your blessings' because they can't.

What Is Depression?

Depression carried a great amount of stigma in the past, so it's only in recent years that people have begun talking openly about the mental illness. Before someone who is diagnosed with depression can hope to function normally again, their condition needs to be treated with either counselling or medication – after all, depression is an illness.

Someone with depression will find that they are no longer interested in activities that once brought them joy. They'll feel isolated, cut off from other people, and sad.

Depression can result in an inability to function sexually, focus on studies, take part in family activities and social life, or get any work done. Unsurprisingly, all of this will have a detrimental effect on the person's life.

There isn't always a specific cause for depression, though in some cases it can be triggered by a traumatic event like getting fired, a serious accident, bereavement or divorce. For example, post-partum depression is triggered by childbirth. A family history of depression can be enough for someone to develop the illness. However, in physical terms depression is caused by an imbalance in the brain chemicals that affect mood and sense of well-being.

"I lost weight. I could barely make myself eat, get out of bed or wash myself. I seemed to be living in a state of numbness. Other days I felt happy, but felt like an overstretched elastic band. I'd snap back into a temper tantrum at the smallest setback. Once, I even got so angry with my son that I slapped him hard enough to leave a bruise, and I can't even remember what he did that made me so angry.

"I knew that I needed help when I realised that I was acting just like my father had done."

Allen M,

Dopamine and serotonin are the main chemicals involved in our sense of well-being and mood. Dopamine covers our instinctive reactions, cravings, addictions and reward-activated behaviours. Our ability to socialise comes from serotonin, which helps keep us calm and makes us less likely to be impulsive. In a healthy brain, these chemicals are regulated by messages flowing from neurons in the brain, causing them to ebb and flow and balance each other out.

These chemical levels can become unbalanced in the brains of depressed people when these neurons appear to get 'stuck'.

Some people need medications to help the process of correcting this chemical imbalance and coming to terms with their depression. Others find that counselling sessions work best. In many cases, a combination of both talking treatments and medication are necessary.

Symptoms of Depression

If you've experienced two or more of these symptoms in the last month, you may have depression. The best first stop is to see your general practitioner and make sure you get a check up to eliminate any possible underlying physical health problems that may be causing your symptoms.

- You feel like you're worthless and can't do anything right.

- You have started to overeat, or have lost your appetite even for foods you enjoy. You may now feel guilty or bad about yourself as this may have led to weight gain or weight loss.

- Even though you aren't any more active than usual, you feel tired all the time.

- You're struggling to keep your home tidy or to take care of your own personal hygiene. Your sex drive is very low.

- You've started feeling like you'll never achieve anything, and that there's no point in trying. You may have feelings of despair and pessimism.

- Little things have started to irritate or annoy you very easily, and you've started having mood swings.

- Your sense of humour has deserted you and you feel like you'll never be happy.

- You find yourself thinking about death a lot, and suicide.

- You feel generally unwell, non-specific aches and pains, headaches or upset stomach, yet you can't pinpoint a reason for these.

- You aren't interested in your everyday activities, including those that you normally enjoy.

- You have feelings of anxiety, sometimes intense, but can't identify a reason.

- You take a long time to fall asleep, or sleep comes easily but you wake up in the night and can't get back to sleep. Or you are sleeping much longer than normal, and find it hard to get up at the proper time.

> "While many new mums report feeling tearful and unable to cope at times, and feeling tired while having trouble sleeping, a woman with post-partum depression may also feel very inadequate, unable to concentrate, unable to enjoy activities, have a poor appetite or compulsive overeating, and have thoughts of suicide."

* The list above isn't intended as a tool for self-diagnosis – your medical practitioner is the best person to make a proper diagnosis of depression and suggest treatment.

You should seek professional help if you are experiencing symptoms like these, and they're lasting more than a couple of weeks. Your doctor will listen to your symptoms and suggest a treatment if they deem it necessary. Your doctor can also advise you about counselling and what facilities are available in your area.

Common Forms of Depression

There are a number of different types of depression, though the most commonly diagnosed form is clinical or major depression. Aside from clinical depression, "manic depression", more commonly known as bipolar disorder, postpartum depression and SAD (seasonal affective disorder) are the three most common types.

Although the causes of these conditions can be different, they tend to have similar symptoms.

Postnatal Depression

After giving birth, up to 80% of new mothers report feeling sad, depressed, or having a low mood. This is sometimes known as the "baby blues". With childbirth regularly described as one of life's happiest events, it's common to be upset or scared if the process ends up leaving you with negative emotions. Some parents end up worrying that they won't be able to love their child, and others feel alone, embarrassed or afraid that they won't be able to cope with the responsibility for this tiny new life.

The good news is that these feelings pass very quickly in most cases, usually lasting no longer than five days. If it seems to be continuing longer than this, it's worth talking to your doctor about it.

Postpartum non-psychotic depression, also known as postnatal depression, is much more serious however. Although lots of new parents feel unable to cope at times, don't get as much sleep as they need and feel tearful, people with postnatal depression may also have thoughts of suicide, and generally feel very inadequate, detached, have a poor appetite or compulsive eating, and difficulty concentrating. These feelings interfere with her ability to look after the baby and bond with her.

Some parents with postnatal depression will live in fear of accidentally harming their new child, and may worry unduly about their baby's health and wellbeing.

Some parents with postnatal depression will be extremely scared of what will happen to their child if they die, and in extreme cases their suicidal thoughts may extend to considering killing their child. Parents experiencing these feelings should contact their health visitor or GP to get help immediately. It's important to have support at this time, even though these irrational thoughts are rarely acted upon.

The rare condition postpartum psychosis is more serious still. It occurs within three weeks of birth, and sees the new parent experience hallucinations, changeable moods, sleeplessness, delusions and agitation. Again, it is very important if you or someone you know is experiencing these feelings, that you seek medical help. Parents with this very severe form of depression may actually act on their thoughts of hurting themselves or their child, while convincing health workers that everything is fine.

Adjustment Disorder

A person may be left feeling depressed, exhausted and unhappy after a stressful experience such as a frightening or upsetting event. For example, being involved in a traffic accident can leave you shaken, uncertain about your own competency, and can result in depression. This type of depression usually passes relatively quickly. The event which resulted in these feelings can easily be linked to the emotions present.

This is your mind's way of coming to terms with what has happened. Adjustment disorder has some symptoms in common with clinical depression, but is much milder.

Winter Depression (Seasonal Affective Disorder)

Wondering if summer will ever come again is very common when we get fed up with winter and are just waiting for the rain and cold to give way to sunshine. It's believed that the lower number of daylight hours, possibly combined with lower levels of naturally occurring vitamin D from sunlight, causes an imbalance in brain chemicals and a usually mild level of depression that can last all winter.

Depression sparked by winter's lack of sunshine is an issue for a surprisingly large number of people, for whom the winter blues can turn into something more serious. For those affected by seasonal affective disorder and seek to alleviate the symptoms, getting outdoors is recommended, along with taking vitamin D supplements, sitting under a sunlamp and exercising.

"Don't brush off that yearly feeling as simply a case of the "winter blues" or a seasonal funk that you have to tough out on your own. Take steps to keep your mood and motivation steady throughout the year."

Mayo Clinic

Bipolar Disorder (Manic Depression)

Thanks to the popular idea that some writers and artists create their best work during manic periods bipolar disorder has been greatly romanticised in fiction. These works are often, in reality, unintelligible to the rest of the world. The artist, when the mood swings into depression, will see the work as vastly disappointing. Sadly, works created during a manic episode often only seem wonderful to the artist while they're in the process of creating them. The sufferer may reach a point of physical collapse because of the heightened activity and sense of achievement during the 'manic' phase.

This form of depression involves mood swings between deep depression and states of euphoria, with some swings lasting days and others only a few hours. A milder form of this illness, cyclothymic disorder, consists of similar but less extreme mood swings.

The name "bipolar" means "both poles" – positive and negative. Suicide attempts may take place in some cases, as the depressive cycle that follows a manic episode can be so severe. The extreme highs and lows of bipolar disorder can be distressing not just for the sufferer but for the people around them.

A person may experience a range of symptoms during a manic episode:

- Intense excitement and joy.
- Grandiose sense of self.
- Difficulty sleeping or winding down.
- Impulsiveness.
- Reduced inhibitions and higher risk-taking.
- Planning grandiose schemes without seeing them as unrealistic.
- Fast speech and movement.
- A high level of creative ideas.
- Irritation with people who don't share this feeling.

Some patients may also experience psychotic symptoms like unreasonable frustration at being unable to carry through creative ideas, hallucinations, delusional thinking and disconnection from reality.

Counselling and medication can fortunately be used to treat this illness once it is diagnosed.

Persistent Depressive Disorder (Dysthymia)

Often going undiagnosed, persistent depressive disorder, or dysthymia, is another form of depression which can last for years. Once diagnosed, dysthymia can be treated, usually by psychotherapy.

This longevity of the illness and its low level leads to people assuming the low energy, lack of optimism, etc, is actually a normal part of the person's personality. Often persisting over a period of years, people with this condition can experience low level depression which lasts for a very long time. Reaching the highest level of their ambitions, talents and skills can be impossible for people with dysthymia, as their low level depression creates a dysfunction which saps all of their motivation.

Therapy to treat dysthymia may be enhanced with a course of antidepressant drugs if there has been no noticeable improvement after three months.

Creative Depression

Creativity is very much possible in those with depression, so we'll end this chapter on a positive note. Before inspiration can strike, some writers, artists and other creative people whose work strongly hinges on mood emotion claim that a period of creative "down" time is necessary. So, perhaps depression has a good side to it for some people!

Certainly the period before starting a new project may seem to be a very quiet and lethargic time for some artists; sometimes to the point where they may actually despair that they'll ever be inspired again. Maybe it's the case that the subconscious mind needs the conscious brain to take a "time out" so that it can cook up some new creative ideas.

Certain artists have reported that after a period of depression they may just wake up one morning with a renewed sense of enthusiasm for their work, and that once they enter the creative zone they're then able to produce work that their subconscious seems to have almost fully developed.

"Some artists, writers, and other creative folk who are traditionally considered to be mercurial in their moods claim to actually experience a creative 'down' time before inspiration hits."

Summing Up

- Affecting as many as one in five people at some time in their lives, depression is one of the world's most common mental health conditions.

- Even the most ordinary routines in life can become almost impossible to someone with depression. These people might lose interest in the projects and pastimes that once brought them the most joy, retreat from social contacts, miss days at work or have difficulty fulfilling their regular duties.

- Some people with depression find that they have nothing that they enjoy, no reason to get up in the mornings and nothing to look forward to. They may feel that they are not really connecting with the people around them, that they are worthless, do not deserve the few good things they have and that there is no meaning to life.

- You are twice as likely to suffer from depression if one of your parents suffers from the illness.

- It's not all bad news, however!

- In order to avoid or reduce future bouts of depression, experts generally agree that a combination of antidepressants and talking treatments is the best way to make sure that people with depression can recover and develop all the coping tools they need.

- There are a number of ways of treating depression, from counselling or psychotherapy to get to the root cause of the problem, to drugs that will help raise the person's mood and get them back to being able to cope with life again.

- Many people today are reluctant to take drugs, especially if it's going to be long term medication.

- Children as young as pre-teen have been diagnosed as depressed, and if the first onset of depression occurs early in life there is a much greater chance that other occurrences will follow.

- Depression can hit at any age.

- Many depressed people say they feel intense sadness, and feelings of being totally alone and unloved.

- Everyone feels blue or down at some time, but when these feelings are intense and go on for a long time without any apparent reason, then perhaps it's time to consider whether or not you are clinically depressed.

2

Why Do People Develop Depression?

Triggers

Just as there are millions of people out there who are experiencing depression, there are potentially just as many answers to the question "What causes depression?" There is no one-size-fits-all explanation, as helpful as one would be. However, with some thought many people diagnosed with depression can often pinpoint some trauma or stressful life event that occurred before they became ill. Many of life's events are stressful even when they are joyful – childbirth, for example.

Here's a list of some of the events that may trigger a depression reaction:

- Death of a loved one.
- Giving birth.
- Divorce, separation or relationship issues.
- Death of a pet.
- Getting a new job or moving to a different office.
- Getting attacked or robbed.
- Substance abuse.
- Money troubles.
- Poor body image.
- Ageing and menopause.
- Winter blues.
- Abusive childhood in the past or abusive relationship in the present.
- Certain prescription medications – always check with your doctor.
- An accident, even if there is no serious injury.
- Loneliness or loss of friends.
- Moving house.
- Physical illness or chronic pain.
- Marriage.
- Unemployment.

Can you add your own triggers to this list for discussion with your doctor, therapist or a close friend?

Changes in the brain chemical balance can occur for obvious reasons in some people, while in others it will seem as though there is no identifiable trigger. Some people do appear to be more vulnerable to depressed moods than others, however, and some biochemical changes can be identified. It's just that, because of personal background, experiences, genetics, or something that science hasn't yet pinpointed, some people are more likely to become depressed than others.

You may be more likely to be diagnosed with depression if a close relative has experienced the illness, for example. A genetic factor may be the cause here, or it may be due to proximity. Scientists say this may be due in part to an inherited gene called 5-HTT, which affects the levels of serotonin in the brain. And no matter what the movies might suggest, you don't have to go through a terrible trauma or have a damaging upbringing to develop depression.

If you want to ward off the possible side effects of happy occurrences that carry a high stress factor – things like getting married, getting a promotion at work or a new job, and buying a new home – it's wise to pay extra attention to a healthy lifestyle with good nutrition and to get plenty of exercise and sleep.

Your depression may be caused by a single factor, a number of unrelated factors or a number of factors that are interlinked.

What Makes Someone Vulnerable?

At some point in their lives, everyone is vulnerable to depression. People most vulnerable to depression are those who may have:

- Experienced depression before.
- A family history of depression, or close relatives with the illness.
- Grown up in a household with one or more depressed parent(s).
- Anyone whose wife, partner or close relative is suffering from depression.
- Have had low level depression for some period of time (dysthymia).

"I was tired all the time, and wasn't interested in anything. A friend said I might be depressed, but I couldn't imagine why I should be. I regret that now – all that time when I was unhappy and made those around me unhappy.

"Something was wrong with me, I was sure of it. I was crying all the time. But there was no reason to – my marriage was going great, I had an amazing job and a nice home. My husband eventually insisted I see a doctor when I started having thoughts of suicide. It turns out depression just happens sometimes. You don't have to be poor or lonely or unemployed or have experienced a trauma. It can happen anyway.

"My doctor prescribed drugs and with the support of my counsellor, I finally started living again."

Beth G.

Typical depressed thoughts:

- I have no purpose.

- I am a terrible employee/guardian/friend/partner.

- I am unintelligent.

- I never learn from my mistakes.

- Life isn't worth living.

- I never get anything right.

- I'm not very attractive.

- I'm not likeable and have no friends.

Further episodes of depression will always be a possibility for anyone who has experienced depression in the past.

Some people believe that people can avoid further occurrences or prevent themselves from becoming depressed in the first place just by changing their attitude. The idea is that you will be less likely to become depressed if you manage to train yourself to think positive, rather than negative thoughts. This is known as Learned Optimism.

It's also possible, with negative thinking, for your thoughts to become self-fulfilling. This kind of thinking becomes a self-fulfilling prophecy as you give up trying to move forward with your ambitions because you think you don't have what it takes, so why bother?

Optimistic thoughts might include things like…

- I try my best to be a good person.

- Being a good employee/guardian/friend/partner is really difficult, but I'm trying my best.

- I'm not stupid – everyone has their strengths and weaknesses.

- I know how to learn from my mistakes and move on with my life.

- Life has its good times – I just have to hang on till it gets better.

- When I look at the good things in my life, I realise I must have done some things right!

- I may not be a great beauty, but I make the most of what I have and besides, looks aren't everything.

- I may not have a lot of friends, but the ones I have really like and support me.

These upbeat thoughts of optimism may sound a little "corny" at times, but there's a big difference between them and more typical negative, depressed thoughts.

"I don't have what it takes to be successful. I wasn't good enough for the job I wanted." would be a common negative response to missing out on a job you applied for, for example. More constructive thinking is: 'I didn't get the promotion, but the competition was strong. I'll continue to improve my skills so I'll do better next time.'

If you respond to this situation with negative thoughts and become resigned to a job you don't like because you think it's the best you can do, you'll appear disinterested and unmotivated to your bosses and co-workers, don't do your best work, and will find it even more difficult to find a job that makes you happy. If it sounds a bit like a Catch-22 situation, that's because it is. But with proper intervention, the cycle doesn't have to go on forever.

Of course, in many cases of clinical depression simply practising positive thinking will not be enough to "get rid" of your depression, but it may be a useful tool that you can try alongside professional medical treatment.

How Family History Can Determine Your Risk Factors

"People experiencing depression do have lower levels of some neurotransmitters – the chemicals that carry brain messages between neurons – such as serotonin and dopamine. What isn't yet fully understood is the cause-and-effect cycle: does being depressed cause the chemical imbalance, or does the chemical imbalance cause the depression?"

Your risk of becoming depressed is higher if you have a family history of depression. It appears that, following a triggering life event, you are more likely to become depressed if you have inherited the gene 5-HTT which alters the amount of serotonin you have. Also, because we tend to model ourselves and our attitudes on those of our parents, we may also unconsciously pick up on the negative thinking that we see them demonstrate.

Dopamine and serotonin, which are neurotransmitters which work to carry brain messages between neurons, are found in lower levels in people who are experiencing depression. Whether this chemical imbalance is causing the depression or caused by the depression remains to be seen, however.

Let's return to that serotonin-affecting gene 5-HTT. A genetic predisposition for depression may exist in the children of parents with depression, owing to the fact that we inherit our genes from our parents. There's no hard and fast rule, however. Not everyone who experiences depression has a family history of the illness, and not everyone who doesn't have the family history is immune to depression. Like so many other possible genetic inheritances, this is a game of chance.

Life Change Units

Back in the 1960s Drs T H Holmes and R H Rahe carried out groundbreaking research into the stress levels of various life events, and gave each event a number of points which they called Life Change Units. To come up with a rough estimate of the amount of stress someone has experienced, researchers Holmes and Rahe developed a stress scale in which events in a person's life in the previous year are assigned Life Change Units which can then be added up.

According to Rahe and Holmes, if you've accumulated more than 200 life change units in the past 12 months, you may be at risk of illness.

If you have scored 300 or higher, you are at risk of illness. If you've scored between 150 and 299, you have a slightly lower risk of illness (around 30% lower than the previous group). If you have scored less than 150, your risk of illness is low.

Rahe and Holmes theorised that a person's risk of developing certain mental health issues, such as depression, is increased based on the number of Life Change Units they had experienced in the past year.

It's worth noting that this list includes a number of seemingly positive events – such as holidays and promotions. Although these seem like happy events on the surface, they do carry the potential for family strife and instability.

Life Event	Mean Value	Life Event	Mean Value
Death of a spouse	100	Divorce	73
Marital separation from mate	65	Imprisonment	63
Death of a close family member	63	Major personal injury or illness	53
Marriage	50	Being fired at work	47
Marital reconciliation	45	Retirement from work	45
Change in the health of family member	44	Pregnancy	40
Sexual difficulties	39	New family member (i.e. birth, adoption, family member moving in, etc)	39
Business readjustment	39	Major change in financial state (i.e. a lot worse or better off than usual)	38
Death of a close friend	37	Changing to a different line of work	36
Change in frequency of arguments	35	Taking on a mortgage (for home, business, etc …)	31
Foreclosure of mortgage or loan	30	Major change in responsibilities at work (i.e. promotion, demotion, etc)	29
Child leaving home	29	Trouble with in-laws	29
Son or daughter leaving home (marriage, attending college, joined mil.)	29	Outstanding personal achievement	28
Spouse starts or stops work	26	Beginning or ceasing formal schooling	26
Change in living conditions	25	Revision of personal habits (clothing, associations, quitting smoking)	24
Trouble with boss	23	Change in residence	20
Major changes in working hours or conditions	20	Changing to a new school	20
Change in recreation	19	Major change in church activity (i.e. a lot more or less than usual)	19
Change in social activities	18	Taking on a loan (car, tv, freezer, etc)	17
Change in number of family reunions	15	Holiday	13
Minor violation of law	11		

Summing Up

- Given the right triggers, just about anyone could develop depression.

- Even life changes that are generally considered to be joyful occasions can have a negative impact, as many of these life events can spark a depressive episode. The extra responsibility that a career promotion brings, the birth of a child, moving house and marriage are all common examples of this.

- The difference between coping and becoming depressed can sometimes lie in a person's attitude to life, so it's important to be aware of the effect these changes can have.

- Depression can sometimes be staved off or lessened by a sense of control, and taking control of your responses to things can be a big help.

- Try to recognise where you may be vulnerable and do something about these situations before they become serious enough to leave you feeling depressed.

- Negative triggers can include unemployment, financial problems, bereavement, relationship problems, divorce, difficulties with children and conflicts in the workplace. For example, if your family is complaining that they never see you because you're always too busy, then issues that would be solved in day-to-day interaction can fester and erupt into full-blown conflict, triggering depression.

- Some people are made more vulnerable by family history, previous depressive history, or serious trauma.

- In properly trained hands, hypnosis is a valuable tool which can help a person remember past incidents and feelings, and perhaps reveal the root of problems; for example, it is often used for phobias.

3

You're Depressed – What Now?

Now that you have a diagnosis, you will have to start making some informed decisions about the treatment that's right for you, in consultation with health professionals. You probably have a mixture of feelings: relief that you know there really is a problem and it's not a more serious physical ailment; glad that you're not lazy or weak; anxiety about how people will relate to you if they think you have a mental illness; fear that you're never going to feel any better.

Talking to your doctor about the way you feel took a lot of energy and strength, but you've finally done it. You are depressed, and you aren't sure what to do with that diagnosis. The time has come to choose what you're going to do about treatment, and this is something that's likely to cause even more confusion. It's hard to know what will actually make you feel better.

Will talking to a therapist really work? Are medications a good idea? Whether it's a consultation with a counsellor or your GP or a heart-to-heart with a loved one, it's important to seek help now. Input from someone else can really help put things into perspective when you're making this sort of decision. You can also benefit from building a support network with friends who know you suffer from depression and who will support you in a 'buddy system' when you're feeling down.

"Please remember that your counsellor isn't an agony aunt; they're not there to give you advice but to work with you so that you are empowered in the knowledge of your problems and able to find your own answers."

"No one ever called it depression when I was growing up because it was associated with mental illness and that was a stigma back then. My mother had 'low moods' and my grandfather was 'bad with his nerves'. I felt ashamed when I grew older and started having the same mood swings I'd seen in them growing up. I put off going to the doctor or seeking any kind of help for years.

"Eventually, I met with a therapist and they suggested I might have depression. Having it out in the open was such a relief. Depression isn't anything to be ashamed of. I'd really advise anyone going through that not to be afraid to talk about their feelings, and to get help if they need it. You can get help to treat this. It's an illness, just like any other."

Harry O.

Counselling or Medication?

Life would be so much easier if there was a one-size-fits-all solution, but there isn't. Each person's treatment needs are different because, as we have already discussed, depression is different in each person.

Your doctor is the best person to talk to if you have any concerns about antidepressant medications, and will be able to give you some good advice. You can also do your own research and seek out depression support groups. In-house counselling services are available in certain doctor's surgeries.

The Role of Therapy

Often called 'the talking therapy', counselling encourages you to look at the personal issues behind your depression. This helps to give you a new slant on things. Counselling can be very helpful for some people, especially if they suspect there is some past trauma in their life or if they know there is a recent triggering event that has sparked their depression.

The goal is to find your own solutions to the issues bothering you by talking to a counsellor and trusting their support.

It's important to keep in mind that a counsellor is not an agony aunt. Their job is to work with you to create the tools you need to understand your problems and find your own answers, not to give you advice and solve your problems for you. When you say something to your counsellor, they're likely to repeat it back to you in a slightly different way. This is known as 'reflecting', and is one of the key ways a counsellor can help you find your solutions.

It's important that you take your time and find a counsellor you are comfortable talking to. Most counsellors teach their clients relaxation techniques that they can practise at home to improve their general sense of wellbeing and sleep patterns. Two schools of psychological thought come together to create the most common form of counselling available today – CBT, or cognitive behavioural therapy.

This combines behavioural psychology with cognitive psychology. Cognitive means 'knowing' or understanding the reasons why someone feels as they do in order to bring about change; behavioural involves changing, adjusting or learning new behaviours. Psychotherapy can really benefit from this combination. CBT works to help you feel better by figuring out and coming to an understanding of why you feel the way you do, then finding a way to change your behaviour to improve this.

"Most counselling these days is cognitive behavioural; this is based on two schools of psychological thought. One is cognitive psychology, the other is behavioural psychology."

An Example of Reflecting

Client: I think I started feeling depressed around the time my mother moved in with us.

Counsellor: Do you think you're depressed because your mother lives with you?

Client: Yes, I think so.

Counsellor: Why do you think that's happening?

Client: Hmm, well there's an extra mouth to feed for one thing.

Counsellor: And this creates a financial burden that is making you depressed?

Client: I don't actually mind the extra work and expenses really, I love my mother. It's just that she's so unwell right now.

Counsellor: And you're feeling depressed because you have to see your mum so ill?

Client: Yes, it's really difficult.

Counsellor: That makes sense. Watching someone you care about go through a serious illness can be quite painful.

Client: Yes. It's so scary sometimes.

Counsellor: What is it that scares you so much?

Client: I'm not even sure – that's the silly thing.

Counsellor: Not at all! Why would being afraid be silly?

- Silence -

Client: I'm scared that she's going to die soon and I'll be all alone. I don't know what I'd do without her.

In this exchange, the counsellor is able to encourage the client to dig deep and discover that their fears of losing their mother are causing their depression, and not simply the extra work and money it takes to care for her.

To help a client dig deeper into their subconscious, some counsellors may even recommend they try hypnotherapy. Your hypnotherapist will explain to you that hypnosis cannot make you do anything you wouldn't want to, or would consider embarrassing or unethical. The word "hypnosis" will often bring to mind embarrassing behaviours like clucking like a chicken as part of a corny stage act, but this is not something to worry about.

Hypnotherapy is a much more respectful, gentle procedure. Counsellors will generally refer their client to a trusted colleague, though some may be trained in hypnotherapy themselves.

Counselling can be quite expensive but it may be covered under some health schemes, and many companies include counselling sessions in their employee health insurance plans. Some counsellors offer a free first time meeting – not a counselling session but time for the two of you to meet and see if you're a good fit. Keep in mind that a big part of therapy will involve talking about personal things you may have never discussed before, and opening up your life and your feelings.

It's important that you find a therapist who works for you, and this may involve meeting with a number of people before choosing just one. You may even find that a friend can recommend someone. You can look in the telephone directory to find counsellors who work in your area, or your doctor can recommend one or more counsellors that they think will suit you. You can usually also get information from health clinics.

How Do I Know Which Counsellor to Pick?

When choosing a counsellor, don't be afraid to ask questions and keep the following points in mind:

- Is there a waiting list, or will you be able to get an appointment soon? Remember that some counsellors have very busy practices. Will they be able to offer you an appointment at a time of day that suits your schedule?

- Is it affordable? How much do they charge per session?

- You have every right to ask about credentials – it's your health and your money, after all!

- What type of therapy do they offer? Is it suited to your needs? Ask them to explain it simply to you.

- Do you feel comfortable with this counsellor? Do you feel they let you speak freely without interrupting you? Do you feel they reflect back correctly what you are saying?

- If cost is a problem, do they have a sliding scale of fees geared to income?

- Is the counsellor accredited in a way recognised by your medical insurance provider?

It is important that you feel safe with this person and that you are sure confidences will not be betrayed. Counsellors will not be able to give you the names of their other clients as references for you to speak to, so asking for references is problematic. Confidentiality plays a major role in all legitimate counselling practices. However, there may be some occasions when you will want your counsellor to speak to your doctor or another health professional, and many counsellors will ask you to sign a waiver to allow that to happen should the need arise.

Many therapists will stress to their clients at the first meeting that anything said in their room will stay in that room. No one except you and your counsellor will know what you say, whether you cry, laugh, get angry or say things that embarrass you or make you feel guilty.

The Role of Medicine

There's no doubt that once you settle on the right drug and the right dosage, antidepressant drugs do work for most people. Some drugs will work better for one patient than another, and this is understandable when you consider how different depression may be from one person to another and the differences in brain chemical imbalances.

This is why so many different drugs have been developed to help with depression.

We are yet to figure out exactly why antidepressant drugs are effective, in the same way that the causes of chemical imbalances in the brain still aren't properly understood. Since the late 1950s, antidepressant drugs have been used to treat depression.

Antidepressant drugs come in several different classes:

- Imipramine and amitriptyline, which are tricyclic drugs (TCAs).

- The most commonly prescribed form of antidepressant is the selective serotonin reuptake inhibitor (SSRI), which was developed in the 1980s. Celexa, Prozac, Paxil, Luvox and Zoloft are just some of the brand names these medications are sold under.

- The newest class is the reuptake inhibitors which block the reuptake of different neurotransmitters (brain chemicals). Serotonin and norepinephrine reuptake inhibitors are becoming popular. (SNRIs)

- Monoamine oxidase inhibitors (MAOIs). There are three types of MAOIs, phenelzine, sold as Nardil, and isocarboxazid and tranylcypromine, sold as Parnate. A third is moclobemide, a reversible MAOI, which acts by reversing inhibition.

One thing to bear in mind is that most health professionals would recommend that a client take both antidepressant drugs and counselling. While drugs can make the patient feel better quite quickly, working with a counsellor can help resolve the issues surrounding the onset of the depression and perhaps prevent a future recurrence. Your doctor will discuss these antidepressant drugs with you, and outline any possible side effects.

The latest antidepressants, SNRIs, appear to have fewer side effects than the earlier ones. The issue of side effects is one of the main concerns surrounding any drug which works in the brain. You should also know that some antidepressant drugs should not be mixed with certain foods.

"In the same way that the causes of the chemical imbalances aren't properly understood, so the reasons that antidepressant drugs work are also not fully known."

Serious risk of overdose is least likely in SSRIs, so they are prescribed most frequently despite their slightly higher risk of side effects.

Foods like red wine, cheese and fermented soy products like Marmite and Bovril should all be avoided by anyone taking MAOIs, as they all contain tyramine.

Do not be afraid to ask questions when your doctor is discussing these medications with you. Depression is often triggered by a past or current trauma or stressful event, even though the depression as a whole is caused by a brain chemical imbalance. This is why most health professionals now agree that for treatment of depression to be effective, it is necessary to treat the causes as well as the symptoms.

So it makes sense that most doctors recommend a combination of counselling and medication. In addition, counselling aims to help the client develop coping strategies – the behavioural part of cognitive behavioural therapy – which will empower them to recognise and avoid triggers in the future. Counselling may even prevent a relapse by helping you sort out the issues that caused the depression in the first place – though antidepressants can be prescribed if you do have a relapse into another episode of depression.

While another episode of depression is always possible, counselling can provide you with the tools you need to manage and recognise warning signs before your depression has a chance to become a serious issue. Here are some tips that may come in handy if you are taking antidepressants:

- Make sure you know what your medication is called and what it's supposed to do, and talk to your doctor about the possible side effects.

- Unexpected and sometimes dangerous side effects may occur if you take two or more medicines that interact with each other. Double check all new prescriptions with your chemist or pharmacist, and make sure your doctor knows if you are taking any other medicines.

- Your pills will come with an instruction leaflet – read it. Call your doctor's office straight away if you feel unwell or suspect you are experiencing an adverse reaction or side effect from the drug.

- Never take anyone else's medications or let them take yours.

- Remember that alcohol and antidepressants don't mix and can even be a dangerous combination.

- Never change the dosage of your medicine, or stop taking it altogether, without first talking to your doctor.

- Sometimes herbal medicines, vitamin supplements, and dietary variations, for example being on a gluten-free diet, may have an effect on the effectiveness of your medicine. Again, check with your doctor.

- Take the medicine exactly as prescribed, for maximum effectiveness.

What Can I Do to Make Things Better?

"Always have something to do that you enjoy; start a hobby, or join a club, take a class. This gives you a reason to get up in the morning and encourages you to socialise and build a circle of friends."

400 people who had not been diagnosed as depressed and 400 people who were beginning treatment for depression were compared in a study by Andrew Billings and colleagues in 1983. The idea that depression usually has a trigger was supported by their findings:

Compared to the non-depressed group, the depressed group had experienced twice as many losses, such as a bereavement, unemployment, loss of income or divorce in the previous year.

Those in the depressed group tended to have fewer family members or friends willing to give emotional support.

The depressed group had relatively more sources of long term psychological pressure, such as a medical condition, family conflict, or workplace stress.

10 Things You Can Do to Help Yourself

There are a number of ways that you can improve your own chances of easing depression and avoiding a recurrence. These include…

1 Be kind to yourself. Get plenty of fresh air and exercise, look after your health, avoid getting overtired and eat nutritious food.

2 Create a support network. Make sure you have an understanding friend that you can call or meet for a chat and a coffee when you're feeling a bit down. Let those who care about you know that you suffer from depression, and build on those relationships.

3 Think of the things you can feel grateful for, and use these to make a list of the good things in your life. Go back to this list as often as you can. Your life may well be much better than you think it is!

4   Use positive statements to override those little voices that whisper negative things in your ear. Try to remain positive and optimistic.

5   Avoid blaming yourself, and understand that it's normal and healthy to feel sad when you experience a loss. Be gentle with yourself.

6   Know when you need help, and don't be afraid to ask for it.

7   Avoid recreational drugs and alcohol.

8   Realise that you are not responsible for anyone else's behaviour.

9   Learn to recognise triggers. Does family conflict bother you? Try to solve problems before they become full-blown conflict. Do you have a toxic work colleague? Arrange your work so that you have as little contact as possible with this person, and make yourself believe that this person's mean behaviour should not be taken seriously.

10 Do things that make you happy. Take a class, start a hobby or join a club. This will help you to build a circle of friends, encourage you to socialise and give you a reason to get up in the morning.

Moving Forward

Work-Life Balance

Are you putting in many more hours at work than you spend with your loved ones? No matter how much you love your job, you still need time for yourself, your family and friends, otherwise you can become jaded, lose interest in your work, and become depressed. One way or another, all work and no play makes Jack – or Jill – pretty miserable.

Does a long commute to your job mean wasted hours, an early start and returning home too exhausted even for conversation? Spending too much time working and not enough enjoying life can bring about depression in a number of ways, including stress induced by overwork. The social support group of your friends who would otherwise help you stave off depression may stop calling you because you're always too busy with work to relax and kick back with them – or even worse, to listen and support them when they need you – and pretty soon you can find yourself isolated.

"Some people immerse themselves in work out of sheer ambition but others do so in order to avoid facing problems in their lives, problems that don't go away and that will eventually scream to be dealt with."

While some people become absorbed by their work out of an impulse to get ahead in life, others will do so as a way of avoiding the problems they face in their personal lives. These problems won't simply go away, however, and will eventually require even more attention than they did initially. Try and get a perspective on your work and remember that, no matter how ambitious you are, you need time to relax and unwind so that you can return to work refreshed and energised.

In order to keep up with a demanding and hectic modern life, many people spend more, rather than less, time working, and even skip the holiday time they desperately need to stay healthy.

Consider learning a new skill just for the self-development, and think about how your family and friends feel when you're never around. As an exercise this week, try keeping a diary of how you spend your time. Are you giving yourself the time you need to think about your life, enjoy a hobby, exercise, relax or just enjoy your own company?

It's time to take control of your life again if you do not currently have the balance you need. Your life can easily become one-dimensional if you do nothing but work. If you end up with no-one to enjoy it with, what's the point in spending all of your time trying to earn money?

10 Ways to Rebalance Your Life and Cut Out Stress

1 Even if you only go as far as the water cooler, take breaks when you're working. Get up from your desk or wherever you're working, and go for a short walk.

2 Rather than working late, organise your workload by priority and be firm in putting the least important jobs off for the next day.

3 Finish work early if you can. Consider delegating some of your workload or share some of the mundane jobs with a colleague.

4 Move closer to work or try to find a job closer to your home if commuting is adding long hours to your workday.

5 Remember that holidays are not a luxury. Set aside time to spend with people whose company you enjoy and find supportive, whether they are family or friends.

6 Learn to leave work at work. What's the point of making time for your loved ones when work issues bleed into it and distract you?

7 Are there any tasks at home or at work that you do out of habit and maybe don't need to do? Ask yourself if there is a way you can drop these time-eaters, or find a more efficient way to clear them up.

8 If possible, give yourself a day off every few weeks, call it a 'mental health' day, and you'll return to work revitalised. If you can't take a day, at least try to leave work a couple of hours early.

9 Block out time on your calendar for a meeting with yourself, while you plan your work and allot time for what you need to do.

10 Go out for lunch, even if it means a packed lunch in the park. Sitting in the sun will boost your vitamin D intake, a natural antidepressant.

Nutrition and Exercise

Exercise releases endorphins, brain chemicals often called the feel-good chemicals for their effect on the way we feel. As well as improving your health and looks, a brisk walk outside, a kick-about game of football or 30 minutes in the gym can really help lift your spirits.

A balanced diet with fresh fruit and vegetables, easy on the junk food and little or no alcohol will help maintain good health and a positive attitude. Eating properly is essential to feeling healthy in mind and body. Give some thought to your diet. Your brain chemicals may actually balance out more easily if you get essential minerals and vitamins from certain foods.

Food for Thought

- Brain function goes nowhere without omega-3, so try using fishy foods to help beat depression. Salmon, anchovies, sardines and mackerel are full of it!

- Leafy green vegetables, whole grains, chicken, bananas and avocados are all great sources of important B-complex vitamins.

- Brain cells, which are called neurons, are like the cells in the rest of your body in that they need protein to build and repair themselves and to function properly, so add meat, grains, vegetables, legumes and tofu to your diet.

- A moderate intake of carbohydrates boosts your serotonin levels and helps lift depression. We're not talking white flour, sugar, cakes and sweets here, which will simply make you heavier, but complex carbohydrates such as whole grain bread, pasta, and cereals, along with fruit and vegetables. These help maintain a steady level of brain chemicals.

- There are also a number of dietary supplements which may be helpful. Talk to your doctor to see what they recommend and to make sure there's no conflict between the supplements and any medication you are prescribed.

Brain-Unfriendly Foods

- Some people believe that depression can be lifted by alcohol because it makes them feel good. However, this effect is only fleeting, and alcohol has a negative impact on your body's ability to absorb vital nutrients like minerals and vitamins. It's not even a food.

- There are two major ways in which sugar can harm your mental state. Too much of it can cause you to gain weight which can lead to depression as a result of a lowered self-image, and the quick energy boost it gives is quickly followed by a slump which can be particularly bad for someone with depression.

- You might feel that the boost from caffeine makes you feel better, but in the long-term, caffeine can over stimulate the nervous system, making you anxious and worsening depression.

Summing Up

- Your doctor will be able to help you to decide if counselling (psychotherapy), antidepressant drugs or a combination of the two will be the best treatment for you following your diagnosis of depression.

- One third of those who take antidepressant medications will find that they work little or not at all.

- For some people, particularly those with an identifiable trigger for their depression, counselling on its own may help.

- You can improve your own chances of easing depression and avoiding a recurrence in a number of ways.

- It's a good idea to try and recognise any triggers that tend to bring on depressed feelings. This way, you can try to either avoid or solve these problems before they can trigger another episode.

- Antidepressant medications and alcohol can be a dangerous mixture, so it's best to avoid drinking when you're on this treatment. Alcohol is also a depressant, so it's worth cutting back even if you aren't taking medications.

- Try to keep a positive attitude and understand that you can't be responsible for anyone else's behaviour.

- Taking a class to learn something new can be a great way to improve your state of mind, as can taking good care of your health and nutrition, getting a reasonable amount of exercise and fresh air and keeping active with occupations that interest you. Try to make time for coffee, an evening out or an afternoon shopping with a friend.

- Try to make an informed decision about the treatment you wish to receive by weighing the pros and cons carefully.

- Drug treatment programmes can be effective, but it's often recommended that you follow them while also receiving a talking treatment.

- Be aware that antidepressant drugs don't work for everyone – they are effective in more than one third of cases, and partially effective in another third.

4

When Someone You Love Has Depression

Depression reaches out its tentacles to family members, friends, co-workers, and anyone within the orbit of the depressed person. Consider the friends who miss the shared interests and mutual support, and the co-workers who have to pick up the slack when work isn't done because someone is too depressed to show up, and who miss the support and camaraderie of their colleague. Imagine the husband or wife starved of interaction, affection and support.

Depression doesn't just affect the person experiencing it – it's like any other illness in that respect. It is a serious condition with serious consequences.

A child of someone with depression may find that they always have to tell their teacher that "Mum's not feeling well and can't help out" at the school fair or other event. They might want to go out and play in the park with their parent, but the parent will have no energy to do that.

"I tried so hard to please her but nothing ever worked; I thought it was my fault she was unhappy. Other kids' mums played with them and laughed a lot; my mum never played with me. Mum was always tired when I was little, and she cried a lot. I was always worried that she was somehow disappointed in me, that she was crying because she didn't like me.

"It affected all my relationships. I was always scared that nobody would ever love me if even my mother couldn't love me. Realising that I hadn't done anything wrong and that my mother had depression took a very long time."

Helen G.

"Sadly, it's when we are depressed that we most need the understanding of caring people around us, and yet our depressed moods can drive them away."

How You Can Help

Any relationship can suffer when depression is involved. It seems unfair that our depressed moods have the potential to drive away those who care about us, precisely when we need their understanding the most.

- Being loving and supportive is the best thing you can do if someone you care about is depressed. Realise that both of you will benefit from maintaining this relationship, and that withdrawing from them will actually just cause further hurt for all involved. That said, you must also accept that you are not responsible for their happiness or unhappiness.

- Even if the tearfulness and futility of your loved one's depression starts to get you down, it's important that you don't complain or belittle them.

- If they aren't regularly meeting with a counsellor and/or their GP, encourage them to do so. Explain how you feel if the situation really starts getting you down, and ask if they'd be willing to go to a counsellor with you. You may be able to help each other, and a counsellor can suggest ways to do this.

- Look for any changes to their depressed mood, and be vigilant. Don't hesitate to contact a counsellor or GP for advice if you become concerned that their mood is worsening or they are expressing suicidal ideation. If you leave it too long, the situation could become critical. It's far better to sound the alarm early and risk getting it wrong.

- You probably won't be able to avoid getting irritated or frustrated at times, but try to discuss the situation calmly. Work together to find ways of making day-to-day life easier.

- If your depressed loved one is taking medication, make sure they take the right dose at the right time. Offer to pick up renewed prescriptions, etc, so they don't run out of pills.

- Find out the name of the doctor or counsellor they are seeing, and keep the phone number handy in case you need to call for advice.

- Work with your loved one to find constructive ways of helping them come out of the depression, perhaps by pinpointing stressful situations in their personal life or employment and looking for solutions. These situations may act as triggers for depression. For example, if you know this person hates confrontation and yet every time there's a family get-together there's a row, discuss this situation and perhaps avoid going to these events until they feel better.

- Because a depressed person often feels overwhelmed by everyday responsibilities, try if you can to take over some of their daily duties until they are able to carry on.

Accept that you, too, are under stress because of the depression and make sure you get enough 'me' time when you can relax and enjoy some time away, just relaxing, thinking or working on a hobby. Always remember to maintain your own support system. Identify the people you know who you can trust with sensitive information, and ask their permission to vent to them occasionally.

Don't feel guilty. If they know you properly, they will understand that your concerns do not negate the love you feel for your depressed partner. At times it may seem that your depressed partner is lazy, pathetic, selfish or weak, and that their behaviour is screwing up your own life, too. It's not uncommon to find yourself wishing your depressed loved one would just "go away" or "get better already".

It's normal to get frustrated. These feelings are perfectly healthy, so long as you do not allow yourself to take them out on your loved one. Depression is a mental illness and it's not possible to just 'get over it'.

It's easier to continue being a supportive friend or partner if you get to recharge your batteries occasionally with a little 'me time'.

The depression will pass in time and you'll have your life back with the person you love. Your loved one did not choose to be depressed, and it's important to keep this in mind. It may seem like depression is dominating your life, but it will get better and it's important that you get on with your own life as far as possible to reduce the resentment that may build up inside you.

Be aware that people who live with someone who is depressed are likely to experience depression themselves, and children of a depressed parent are up to twice as likely to become depressed themselves.

Five Things NOT to Say!

1 Can't you just get over it, already?

2 I'm tired of dealing with this.

3 There are so many people worse off than you – what do you have to complain about?

4 I'm tired of being around you when you don't make any effort.

5 You're making everyone else miserable, buck up!

No one chooses to be depressed, which is why it's important that you don't make any of the unhelpful comments listed above. Sadly, no matter how much worse off other people might be, someone in the midst of depression can't measure their lives like that. Your loved one's sense of worthlessness will only be made worse if you make them worry that you'll abandon them. People with depression need to know that they are loved. Depression can actually be made worse by the guilt that the person will feel if they're made to deal with this type of statement.

If you are caring for a child who may be showing signs of depression or worry that you are experiencing it yourself, be sure to consult a therapist or doctor.

Removing the Stigma around Mental Illness

- There are support groups available in some areas – ask your local social services department, doctor, counsellor or church group if they know of one for people coping with depression.

- Help your loved one to feel more comfortable talking about their depression by discussing mental illness yourself. By now, we should really be leaving the stigma of mental illness in the past where it belongs. There is no shame in having depression.

- Work with them to see if you can identify situations that trigger depressed feelings, and try to work out solutions.

- Tell people that your partner or loved one is depressed if they ask what's going on. Tell them that you'd appreciate their support as co-workers or friends, and this is a mood disorder that they are doing everything possible to recover from.

- Don't stop inviting people around, or accepting invitations to visit friends. Going out and about may lift the mood for both of you, and if you have children, it may be even more important to keep a normal social and everyday routine.

- If your husband, wife or partner is depressed and you have children do try to explain to them what's happening. Keep it suitable for their age group: often a simple 'Mummy/Daddy is not feeling well and that's why they're being so quiet' will be enough. Children don't have a lot of life experience and tend to jump to the conclusion that they are to blame if their mum or dad is unhappy. They think they've done something wrong, and if someone is too depressed to respond to them warmly they may carry that sense of guilt with them into adulthood unless the situation is explained to them. They need to understand that what's happening is no one's fault and that life will eventually return to normal.

"People find it hard to understand why I don't just snap out of it. People would come around and try to cheer me up if I had a broken leg, because they'd see the big plaster cast and feel sorry for me. As it is though, people just think I'm a big lazy pessimist who doesn't want to be happy because I don't join in anything or try to have fun. Nobody can see my depression.

"I do wish my friends would make the effort to come around sometimes, but I can't blame them for not wanting to visit and spend time with me when I'm this depressed."

Joseph W.

You might find it helpful to talk to other people who are supporting depressed friends or relatives, and your depressed partner will feel better knowing they are not unique in this condition. Support groups can be great for depressed people and their families and friends, as they're an invaluable source of support and guidance.

Summing Up

- The effect of depression is to drive people away. This is a real conundrum, as when someone is depressed they will really need the support of their family and friends.

- Counselling, drug therapy, or both will often be required to treat depression. It is a mental illness and not something that you can just snap out of with positive thinking.

- Trying to maintain a social life for the two of you can be really helpful if you're caring for someone who is depressed, and picking up the extra workload at work or home is also a big help.

- It's important for your children's welfare to explain what is happening in a language suitable for their level of maturity.

- Always remember to stay on top of your own health as well as that of your loved one.

- Ensure that you are getting good nutrition, all the sleep you need and plenty of relaxation, just like your loved one.

- Once the period of depression has subsided, you may well find that you and your loved one are able to enjoy life more than ever before. Understanding depression and working together to get through it could bring the two of you closer together.

- Take time out so that you can visit with friends or enjoy a favourite activity, and don't hesitate to seek help for yourself from a doctor or counsellor if you feel that things are getting you down.

- Studies have shown that people close to someone with depression often experience depressed feelings themselves.

- Even very young children can understand if someone isn't feeling well, and you can work with them to help them see that they have done nothing wrong and done nothing to cause their mum's or dad's sadness.

- Try to encourage your loved one to get out and socialise, eat properly and take their medications as prescribed.

- Non-judgemental support, holding back your own frustration and criticism, and encouraging your depressed partner or friend to seek help and take steps to ease their depression are important.

- If you care about someone who is depressed, try to remember that they can't just pull themselves together or get over it.

5

Depression and Suicide

Suicide was viewed as a sin and a cause for great shame in the past. A conspiracy of silence grew up, where doctors would sometimes pronounce a different cause of death to spare a family more suffering, or shamed families would hide the fact of suicide. If someone committed suicide, their body was relegated to unconsecrated ground outside the churchyard walls, as they were not allowed to be buried in hallowed ground. It is, therefore, depression's darkest side.

By now, of course, we understand that neither the individual who has committed suicide nor their family should be blamed when the worst happens. Society has become more compassionate, and we've come to recognise that cases of suicide can be rooted in pain, suffering, physical illness or anger, but that it usually occurs as a result of mental illness. In all circumstances, risk of suicide may be increased by alcohol or drug abuse, and is increased if there has already been a suicide attempt.

Thoughts of suicide are one of the items listed on the checklist for depression, and many of us have the two concepts strongly linked in our minds. Patients diagnosed with major depression have as much of a 6% risk of suicide over their lifetime, so it makes sense that we rarely think about one without considering the other. The risk of depression is even higher in those suffering from bipolar disorder. Studies suggest they may be more than 15 times more likely to take their own life than the general population.

According to statistics body NHS Digital, at any one time in England, one sixth of the population aged 16 to 64 have a mental health problem. 10% of these individuals also admit to having considered suicide.

The Problem with Suicide

Suicide leaves a legacy of grief and guilt among the people left behind, and is a tragic outcome for anyone who commits or attempts it. Some people are left just too emotionally numb to even feel grief.

"For so long it seemed that we were both running on my "life energy". I repressed my enthusiasm at times because it simply didn't go with his depression.

"I went to bed early that night, and because I was coughing so much I slept in the spare bedroom so I would not disturb his sleep. Making sure my husband took the correct dose of his medication was usually my responsibility, but that day I had the flu and just felt too tired. He died of an overdose that night. Would he have overdosed if I had been well enough to see to his medication and be there?

"I have no idea if he did it on purpose or if it was an accident because he was just so disconnected. He didn't leave a note. I was meant to be the one taking care of things, getting up in the morning, making our breakfast. But I was worn out from the flu, and I inevitably reached a point where I could no longer continue to provide enough life energy for us both.

"It seems as though it was inevitable that it would happen eventually, but it's probably something I'll never know for sure."

Seamus R.

It can often seem like the only option, but it always creates more pain than it ends. The friends and families of someone lost to suicide will often spend the rest of their lives wondering if there were warning signs they could have seen and didn't, or if there was anything else they could have done to save their loved one. There is little that can be done to ease the pain of those who cared about the suicide victim and were unable to help, and many of the warning signs of someone about to commit suicide will only be evident after the fact.

Who's Most at Risk?

Visiting old friends or relatives the person has lost touch with, a sudden change of mood and giving away treasured possessions could all be indicators of a possible suicidal intent. If a person you care about is suddenly intent on "making things right", it could be a sign that they've got a whole new lease on life or it could be a sign that they're trying to tie up their loose ends. In many cases, because the person has made a decision to end their life, they may even seem happier and more relaxed to their friends and family.

Thoughts of suicide, according to some studies, are especially common in those who display impulsive or violent behaviours, are addicted to drugs or drinking, have experienced parental separation or divorce, or who have a close friend or family member who has committed suicide. In addition, the risk of suicide is heightened in people who experienced their first episode of major depression in their teens, people who self-mutilate, people with schizophrenia, and new mothers suffering from severe post-partum depression.

People with postnatal depression are at their highest risk of suicide in the first year following the birth of their child.

As you can see, depression is a component in all these additional factors, so suicidal thoughts should not be taken lightly or dismissed without some follow up with a health professional.

"Suicides come in threes" is a phrase you may hear thrown around. Whether or not the number 3 is accurate, it does appear that – especially if the individual is already depressed – having a close friend or relative who commits suicide, or attempts to do so, can be a trigger for suicidal thoughts.

If you're having thoughts of suicide yourself, now is the time to seek help.

"Frequently, the suicidal person may even seem happier and more relaxed to friends and family, because they have made a decision to end their life."

Common Suicide Risk Factors Include:

- Ongoing or serious physical ailments.
- Past incidences of self-harm or self-destructive behaviours.
- Other mental illnesses such as schizophrenia.
- Having a friend or relative who committed suicide or has tried to.
- A history of alcohol or drug abuse.
- Major depressive episodes.

Warning Signs

Some friends or family members will end up subconsciously ignoring warning signs of suicide because the idea of losing someone they care about to suicide is too appalling to contemplate. But even if you're looking out for them, the warning signs tend to vary from person to person and even those that know the person best will miss the clues until it's too late.

The following are some of the most common symptoms that tend to appear in depressed people who are contemplating suicide:

- Expressing the view that they don't expect to be around for upcoming events, and talking about death often.
- Driving too fast, drinking excessively, taking unnecessary risks and doing other things that are out of character. Doing and discussing things that wouldn't normally be expected from them.
- Attempting to set things right, meeting with friends and family members that they haven't seen in some time or trying to mend old arguments.
- Giving away possessions that they treasure.
- Having no interest in planning for the future or setting up activities.
- Suggesting that their family or friends wouldn't miss them or would even be better off without them.

"The slightest thing, something someone said, whatever, left me feeling hurt and numb. In my mind more than my body, I felt as if everything hurt. I got so that I'd stay in bed and daydream about not waking up in the morning. I knew nobody understood what I was feeling, and it made me feel so alone. Eventually I came to the conclusion that life just wasn't worth the effort anymore.

"It felt like a load had been taken off my shoulders once I'd finally made that decision, funnily enough. I met with my friends and they said that I seemed more relaxed and cheerful than they'd seen me in a long time. We actually had a really great time. At the end of the night, I climbed into my car, steered towards a tree and put my foot down. I ended up with nothing more than a bump on the head, though. I hit a wire fence and it stalled my car – just my luck!

"A guy out walking his dog late saw the crash and called an ambulance. I was mad at the time, but now I'm so glad someone saw me and came to help. I just wanted to die at the time, though."

Jane W.

If you're having suicidal thoughts, it's common to feel like the people you care about, maybe even the whole world, will be better off without you. You might feel like you're all alone, and that nobody cares that you're here. Remember that there is help for you and, if you hold on long enough, these feelings will pass. Try your best to take a step back from these thoughts.

Talk to your counsellor, to a close friend or relative, your teacher, school guidance counsellor, company nurse, your family doctor, the personnel officer at work, call the Samaritans or one of the other helplines, tell them how you feel and ask for help. Whatever it takes to get you the help you need – quickly!

Your friends and family will all be devastated if you go now. Exiting their lives by suicide will just leave them with a legacy of grief and guilt, and that isn't what you want for them.

Visit your nearest hospital's emergency department or get someone to take you there, and tell the doctor on duty that you're suicidal if you feel like you're in immediate danger of ending your own life.

The greatest risk of suicide is to be found in people with bipolar disorder. If the individual is using recreational drugs or drinking a lot of alcohol, or they have attempted suicide in the past, this risk is increased further.

How Do I Know if Someone Needs Help?

So what can you do to help someone, when there are so many signs that are so unclear at times? Well, there's a lot you can do to try and stop someone if you think they're considering suicide.

- If someone you care about talks to you about suicide, consider the fact that you may well be the only person you're telling and that this is a cry for help. Even if you promise your friend that you won't tell anyone, don't feel obliged to keep something this big a secret. Express your concern, and talk to other people you trust and who know the person.

- Most people who commit suicide will have expressed their thoughts of dying before they tried to end their lives, so don't fall for the myth that suicidal people don't talk about their plans. There's a strong chance that your friend is raising the subject because they're scared of what they're about to do and want you to stop them.

- Try and get your friend to call one of the many suicide helplines, or to visit their own doctor for help. Get other people to back you in this gentle persuasion. Don't wait and see if it will pass – if necessary, take the person to their doctor yourself.

"If you think someone you know is thinking of suicide, then there's a lot you can do to try to stop them."

What to Do?

- Someone who is considering suicide will already be experiencing enough anxiety, shame and feelings of worthlessness without your judgement, so try to keep your conversation nice and non-judgemental.

- Do not leave them alone.

- Make sure they know that problems can be solved, and that while their feelings are very real now they will pass with time.

- Check their house and make sure they don't have access to things that could be used in a suicide attempt, such as knives, drugs or guns.

- Unless you're a trained mental health professional, understand that coping with suicide needs special skills and do your best to get this help. Understand also that, in the final analysis, if someone you've tried to help goes ahead and attempts suicide, it is not your fault. Don't play the blame game with yourself.

- Even if their words shock you, keep your feelings to yourself.

- Show them you are taking their feelings seriously and that you care about them.

- Persuade them to seek immediate help – either phone the suicide helpline (in the telephone directory) and hand them the phone, or if you think it's urgent, get them to go to the doctor or hospital with you.

Suicide: The Myths

1 **They won't actually do it if they're comfortable talking about suicide.** It's important that you take it seriously if someone you know starts talking about suicide. Many people will talk or hint about suicide first before attempting to end their lives.

2 **Suicidal people will never stop being suicidal.** Most people who consider suicide because they are in a painful situation and this appears to be the only way out. The need to end their life may well go away if they are able to change the situation they are in.

3 **They've already tried and failed to commit suicide once, they won't do it again.** They may well try again if their situation hasn't changed and they've not solved the problems or received medical treatment and counselling.

4 **The type of person who will attempt to end their own life can be easily identified.** There is no single identifiable character type that is more likely to commit suicide than others, though there are a number of warning signs and factors to consider. Just about anyone can experience clinical depression, and this is the most common cause of suicide.

5 **There's no way of knowing if someone will kill themselves.** People who attempt suicide often have a history of mood disorders or life stress difficulties, even if some suicides will appear to be a spontaneous reaction to loss or trauma.

6 **Most suicides follow through without ever asking for help.** Most people considering suicide will have confided their negative feelings in a friend, relative or co-worker. Some may even have visited their doctor.

7 **If someone who's been threatening suicide suddenly seems happier, it means the crisis is over.** It may just mean that they've made a decision to kill themselves, and now feel better as they believe they can see an end to their pain.

8 **Talking about suicide plants the idea in people's minds.** Talking to someone shows you are concerned, and allowing them to talk about their feelings is more likely to help them find another solution or seek help than it is to validate their suicidal feelings.

9 **Someone who wants to commit suicide wants to die.** No, they just want to end the pain, emotional or physical, that they are experiencing. Death may seem to be the only solution to them at that time.

The Controversy of Antidepressant Drugs and Suicide

Antidepressant medications have been used by a significant number of people to attempt suicide by overdose, which is ironic when these drugs are the main treatment of choice by doctors and they work for many depressed people. Researchers are still debating whether, although these drugs are effective in helping depression, they actually help prevent suicide.

The risk appears to be highest in people with previous attempts at suicide, people with a history of self-harm and older people.

Fatal overdoses appear to be less common in those who use SSRIs. An apparent increase in suicide when people started taking SSRIs has largely been dismissed on the basis that people starting medication are newly-diagnosed and in the deepest stages of depression and so more vulnerable to suicidal tendencies. This is one of the reasons that counselling is recommended along with drug treatments as the most effective treatment for depression.

That said, because of concerns raised over a potential relationship between suicidal thoughts and attempts in children and the use of SSRIs, and their tendency to be less effective than some other medications, these are not generally prescribed to young people under the age of 18.

Some experts have theorised that the fact that people start feeling better after taking antidepressants could actually be the cause of any increase in suicidal behaviour among these people. They may well have decided to commit suicide after their depression was lifted by the medication as they have become more capable of making decisions and more aware that their life still has the same problems as before.

It should be noted that there are claims that a number of other drugs besides antidepressants can cause chemical imbalances in the brain. These issues are all undergoing further investigations, so for now the main thing we can take away is that a doctor's directions should always be followed when taking antidepressants, as with all drugs.

The UK government currently requires that every new drug going on sale must require a suicide rating, as chemical imbalances in the brain can be caused by a wide range of treatments for heartburn, hypertension, obesity, acne, insomnia and other conditions.

Information for Kids and Teenagers

Teenagers and young people can often find themselves with a heavy responsibility when their friends talk to them about suicide. Here are some things to look out for if you're worried about a friend's wellbeing.

Does your friend…

- often talk about death?
- avoid mixing and hanging out with friends and relatives?
- drink a lot?
- find it difficult to concentrate?
- do reckless or dangerous things, like speeding?
- experience changes in eating or sleeping habits?
- start using illegal drugs?
- lose interest in their usual activities?
- talk about feeling hopeless or guilty, that life isn't worth living?

Get them to open up and talk about the things that are worrying them. How much do you know about your friend's life and what's going on with them? Have they lost a friend or relative to suicide? They may well be going through something difficult, like the death of a loved one, the break-up of a long-term relationship or parental divorce. Depression and thoughts of suicide could easily be triggered by any of these factors.

What You Can Do

- Someone who is considering suicide can sometimes feel less alone and alienated if they know that someone cares enough to listen to their problems. So listen to your friend. This will also make it easier for you to tell other people who might be able to help, and put you in a position where you can suggest avenues of help for your relative or friend. It can sometimes be hard for depressed and suicidal people to see solutions to their problems, but they might be able to find a way to cope if they are able to talk to someone who listens without judging.

"For the depressed or suicidal person, it can be hard to see solutions to their problems – talking to someone who listens but doesn't judge can help them find other ways to cope."

- Make sure your friend knows that you want to help them find help, that they are not alone and that you care about them. Call the Samaritans and give them your phone. Stay with the person and listen while they talk – sometimes a sympathetic listener can defuse a serious situation and convince a suicidal person to seek help. Encourage them to talk to their parents, and offer to go with them if they need support. Just be there for them. If you're very worried about the person, refuse to leave them on their own until there's someone else there to take over – someone who is qualified to take on the responsibility of helping your friend.

- Seek help from a parent, teacher, school nurse if you're teenagers, or get in touch with the person's doctor or counsellor or some other health professional.

- If your friend doesn't come to you to talk, then open the conversation yourself. Sure, it's not easy to talk about suicide – but it's not easy to be left wishing you'd done something after the fact, either. Be open, tell the person that you're concerned about them, say they seem depressed and talk a lot about death – are they thinking of suicide?

Dealing with a Friend's Suicide

In some cases, people will go ahead and commit suicide even after they receive the support of caring friends and family and the intervention of qualified professionals. If that happens, don't play the blame game – understand that you do not have total control over someone else's actions.

The people who are left behind will be left with a mixture of feelings – from anger that the person has hurt them in this way to guilt that this is in some way their fault.

Some people view suicide as an aggressive gesture, or one that has been made with no consideration for loved ones.

- Talking about what has happened is one way for survivors to help each other. It's important to break through that barrier of silence. Debate why your friend or loved one may have taken their own life, talk openly about what you're feeling now and talk about the person you have lost.

- Say goodbye to the person who has died by holding a ceremony to remember them – provided their family and close friends agree. Agree on a time and give everyone a chance to talk about their memories and feelings.

- Feelings of sorrow and grief are normal, but if you or another person in your group find those feelings aren't fading, it is responsible to seek some help with a counsellor or doctor, or talk to an older family member if you're in a younger age group, and ask for help.

- It might be difficult at this time, but try to share good memories and celebrate your friend's life. Accept that your friend made a decision – not a good one or one you agree with, but a decision nonetheless. It was a decision made out of pain or desperation, and no one is to blame.

Summing Up

- In the past, society had a very unkind view of people who committed or attempted suicide, but we've thankfully grown more compassionate with time.

- It's important to remember that suicide and suicide attempts affect not only the person doing it but also their friends, relatives, and everyone who cares about them.

- Sometimes the indicators that someone was considering suicide are not recognised until after it has happened. Self destructive behaviours like taking drugs or drinking too much alcohol, self-isolation and behaving recklessly, becoming preoccupied with death, giving away treasured belongings, trying to mend old arguments are just some of the warning signs you may spot.

- Many people who are having suicidal thoughts can be helped by skilled intervention, and a lot of suicide attempts are really cries for help.

- It's important that you try to get your loved one to visit their doctor or even the emergency department at your local hospital if they confide their intent to end their own life.

- A threat of suicide really needs the intervention of a qualified health professional, so do what you can and then make sure they get the proper treatment they need.

- Do whatever you can to stop your loved one from attempting suicide. One idea is to call the Samaritans or another helpline on their behalf and then give them the phone. Making the call can be really scary, so taking this first step for them can make a huge difference.

- People, especially young people, often confide their thoughts of suicide to a friend and ask that it is kept a secret – this is one promise that should always be broken.

- There are a number of myths about suicide, such as that someone attempting suicide really wants to die.

- One person's suicide may trigger similar thoughts in others, particularly those who are already depressed.

- Suicide is recognised as the result of deep emotional or physical pain, distress, trauma or mental illness, and it is known that many people who wish to die are suffering from major depression.

- If someone you care about does end up committing suicide, you're likely to experience a wide range of emotions from anger that this has happened to sadness or numbness. Help yourself and your fellow survivors by talking to each other about your feelings and about what has happened.

- Even after you do everything you can, your loved one may well go on to attempt suicide. It happens, and it's nobody's fault.

6

Children Don't Get Depressed, Do They?

Filled with friends, joy, love and games, many of us prefer to think of childhood as a golden time. This idyll isn't truly representative of everyone's childhood, however. Children can't be shielded from every bad thing that happens, no matter how loving their parents, no matter how well-off or sheltered they are. So it's perhaps a fool's paradise to think that children won't experience depression, but this is what was believed for quite a long time.

If you consider that stress is a factor in the triggering of depression, then try to see the world through your child's eyes. Parents divorce, families break up, relatives are lost. They experience the death of their grandparents, and sometimes even their parents. Remember that children don't have the life experience to put these issues into any kind of perspective.

Of course, there are also more terrible things: studies show that as many as one in four children may experience physical or sexual abuse. And to some degree, children will certainly be affected by uncertainty and worries about the future in bad economic times, when jobs are lost and unemployment looms. Our children see these things, too. Abandonment, kidnapping, cruelty and other dreadful things appear in the news every day.

On the Internet and on TV, children see images of death, hurt, war and famine. We now know that these things can have a profound effect on a child's mind. Add to this the fact that even children younger than 10 are being encouraged by the media to be skinny, beautiful, even sexy.

There are a number of studies about the prevalence of depression among children and adolescents. Studies show that children as young as primary level or even pre-school may experience depression.

They're under pressure to be one of the cool kids in the class, while still doing well in all of their exams. There is also our old friend, the 5-HTT gene, which increases the possibility of depression in children who inherit the gene from parents who have had the illness. It's easy to see why depression is more than possible for children when you take all of this into account alongside a whole panorama of world tragedy, pressure from parents, bereavement, a best friend moving away, a difficult teacher, divorce and family discord.

Adolescent girls may be twice as likely to be depressed as adolescent boys. Peer pressure may be the culprit here, with some speculating that the higher rate of depression in adolescent girls could be because of the pressure they are placed under to look like the models and movie stars they see in the media. Add to that all the pressures of adolescence and it's no wonder that some teenagers experience depression.

At any one point in time, it's believed that up to 5% of children and teenagers may be suffering from depression.

Research papers like *Depression and Suicide in Children and Adolescents* by Jellinek and Snyder in Pediatrics in Review.1998; 19: 255-264, and *Depression in Childhood and Adolescence* by Barbara Maughan, Stephan Collishaw and Argyris Stringaris in the Journal of the Canadian Academy of Child and Adolescent Psychiatry (2013) give us a strong insight into what's happening with these young people.

What to Look Out for if You Think Your Child Is Depressed:

1 They have become introverted or reserved, despite normally being outgoing.

2 They have experienced a bereavement, tension in the home or the loss of a parent or close relative or friend. A child may be profoundly affected by even the death of a beloved pet. It may have been a scruffy old dog, a lazy cat or just a goldfish, but if your child loved it, you can bet that they're grieving for it as intensely as an adult would grieve for a human loved one.

3 Depression has affected other members of your family.

4 Teachers have commented that they are troublesome or unfocused in class, or their grades have started dropping.

5 You can't get them up for school in the morning, or they have complained about having difficulty sleeping.

6 They may have started acting out if they are a teenager, and there may be reckless or violent behaviours.

7 They complain about various vague aches and pains, headaches, sore throats, tummy aches, etc.

8 Your child loses their appetite – or seems to eat for comfort.

9 You suspect your child is experiencing bullying at school or in the neighbourhood.

10 You have moved home and your child is missing friends and familiar surroundings.

11 They are usually full of energy but now seem listless.

As you can see, the symptoms of depression in children and teenagers are very like those in adults, and the treatments are both similar and equally successful. The difference is that a child doesn't know what depression is in the way an adult might; and therefore isn't able to tell you that they feel depressed or even sad.

No doubt your doctor or counsellor will give you some advice, but the main points would be to ensure that they take any medication that may be prescribed in the right dosages, and that you are supportive and non-judgemental.

These behaviours may be the result of a number of things, but if your child exhibits one or more of these and they persist for more than a week or so without any change, it's wise to talk to your doctor. It's important to note that this list should not be used to replace a formal diagnosis.

Before discussing the possibilities of depression, your doctor will most likely want to do a physical exam to rule out any underlying health problems. These illnesses include hypothyroid (underactive thyroid gland), diabetes, chronic fatigue syndrome, and multiple sclerosis.

"Try to get your child to talk about things that worry them. Be aware that your child may take very seriously things that you, as an adult, don't consider to be very important."

What to Do Next

If your child has depression, there are things you can do to help them recover. For example, you can avoid making them feel worse if you avoid guilting them with statements like "You have me worried sick" and "This is just like the way Uncle Bill behaved – and look what happened to him!" Try and see the world through your child's eyes.

Your child will be trying to get through whatever has brought on this depression, and this is enough to deal with without having to also worry about their parents being disappointed in them. Perhaps they're getting over the death of a pet. It may be that they are the victim of a school bully, are having difficulties with a teacher or have had a falling out with their best friend.

Perhaps their parents have recently divorced – while this may be a relief to the parents, many children will end up believing that their parents have split up because of something they did, or that they're going to lose whichever parent ended up moving out. If you have recently divorced or separated from your partner, it's a good idea to sit down with your child and your former partner to explain that you both intend to stay in their life despite living apart, that this isn't their fault and that you both still love them. They should make it clear that they love them and that they have nothing to be afraid of.

Encourage your child to tell you about the things they're worried about. Keep in mind that they may well be taking something very seriously that you don't consider very important as an adult. Some children see television coverage of war and violence and become afraid that these things will happen in their town. Their depression may well be caused by something like failing an important test or not getting an academic prize, being embarrassed because they think they aren't developing at the same rate as their peers or not being picked for the sports team.

They may feel that mum's tears or dad's long silences are because they have done something wrong. It's possible you could even have sparked this depression yourself by accident – some parents attempt to encourage good behaviour by talking about kidnappings or murders and suggesting that these things happen if children don't behave.

What may seem like a passing comment to you could easily be fixated upon by a child.

What Should Parents Look For?

Older people and children tend to exhibit very similar signs if they are experiencing depression. Often, a child will say they have vague aches and pains such as tummy ache, headache, or earache, or simply say they feel sick. The child may also stop playing with friends or going to activities or sports they usually enjoy. In some cases, depression may also be a warning signal that the child is a victim of sexual abuse.

Changes in behaviour will often be the first clues you'll see that suggest your child has depression, as they may not have the language or understanding to tell you what they are feeling. Unusually withdrawn behaviour, misbehaviour and arguments with parents and siblings may be indicators of depression in younger children. They may also have unexpected violent outbursts, and another child may end up being bitten or slapped.

They won't have the words or life experience to explain what they're feeling, but they can tell that something is wrong and react to that. A child who was once well-behaved may well become the class troublemaker, and you may even get a call from their teacher to say that their marks have been slipping. Again, going to your general practitioner for a physical check-up is probably the best starting place.

Teenagers may tell you they are unhappy, that they feel down. Teenagers tend to exhibit symptoms more similar to those of depressed adults. Unfortunately, these are behaviours often considered normal for them. They may become generally hard to live with, and be messy, irritable, bad-tempered or withdrawn. A concerned parent should seek professional help, as it may take a professional to figure out whether it's depression or just teenage angst.

You may also notice other warning signs, such as…

- Altered sleeping or eating habits.
- Low energy levels.
- Indecisiveness and poor concentration.

"In younger children, depression may manifest itself in naughty behaviour, in arguing with parents and siblings, or in unusually withdrawn behaviour. Sometimes there are sudden outbursts of violence, such as hitting or biting another child."

CHILDREN DON'T GET DEPRESSED, DO THEY?

- Lower marks and test results, or skipping school altogether.
- Feeling helpless or useless.
- Recurring thoughts of death and suicide, harming oneself.
- Moodiness, irritability, rudeness, aggressive behaviour.
- Difficulty with relationships, social isolation.
- Low self-esteem, feelings of guilt.
- Loss of interest in activities that were formerly enjoyed.

A Different Cause Entirely: Schizophrenia

Despite the popular belief that this is split personality, schizophrenia is actually an acute form of brain chemical imbalance which, with patience and the proper medication, can be eased. Your teenager may be suffering from early onset schizophrenia if their mood swings are extreme and they have started shutting themselves in their room. Be aware of this possibility if they seem to be talking to themselves or having hallucinations, have given up bathing and don't put on clean clothes.

"He got into drink and drugs. He got very anti-social and sometimes wouldn't wash or change his clothes. We thought that standard teenage moodiness were the reason for our son's unpleasant behaviour at first.

"Sometimes we felt like disowning him. It got to the point where our daughters refused to come to any family events if he was going to be there, because he was constantly causing scenes at home. We thought he was either crazy or just plain bad – I know that's a horrible thing to say about your own son, but that's how it was. For no apparent reason, he'd go into these violently angry moods, or he'd start threatening to kill himself.

"It was such a relief when we finally found a doctor who diagnosed him with schizophrenia. It was as though some other horrible person had been living in our son's body, and finally we had the boy we loved back again. We got the teenager we loved back – Sam was gentle and happy again, though it did take some time before they got the balance of medications right."

Conor C.

Treatment for Children with Depression

Antidepressants are sometimes prescribed for children, although many healthcare professionals prefer to try counselling first. Some counsellors specialise in working with children and teenagers, and the majority of young people can be helped with the right form of therapy. Because the child doesn't live in the world alone, most therapists will include the parents and siblings in some sessions, encouraging everyone to speak openly about their problems and to find, with the counsellor's guidance, solutions and accommodations that bring them closer together.

A good counsellor will figure out why the child feels as they do by working with them to determine what initially triggered the depressive episode. They will also work on helping the child to overlay negative thoughts with positive ones, a means of developing a more optimistic and confident outlook on the world. If the child is feeling bad because they're unable to do well at school or don't have a lot of friends, the counsellor will work out a plan to tackle those problems and will also help the child to bolster their self esteem.

The child will be more capable of standing up to bullies and making friends, as they feel more relaxed and able to cope.

"I had a long time girlfriend who mostly I thought I loved but suddenly I wondered if I even wanted to be with her, I felt I wasn't good enough for her. I really wanted to get into university, so I was working really hard at school to get the marks I needed. It felt like there was so much pressure my parents expected a lot of me because I'd be the first to go on to university if I made it.

"But all the while I was terrified my girlfriend was about to break up with me. Without warning, all I could think about was just walking into the sea and it all being over, I just wanted to put an end to it. I was really lucky because I was able to ask if I could talk to my friend's mum, who was a counsellor. Most of all, it was good to talk to someone who didn't judge me or tell me to get over it, but took me seriously.

"After a few months seeing a counsellor and working out some of the issues that had got me down, I started to feel really well. I learned some relaxation techniques, and she helped me understand that there wasn't anything wrong with me, I was just stressed out by all of the pressure."

John C.

Counselling and guidance may also be necessary for other family members as they may be struggling to understand why a normally happy and confident child has become depressed. Try to get everyone to attend, and be as open as possible about family issues.

While teenagers or adults may find medications to be an effective form of treatment, some antidepressants don't work so well on children. Children's brains are still developing, so there's also a degree of reluctance to give young children drugs that affect the balance of chemicals in their brains.

Explaining Depression to Children

A child might not understand why it's important for them to talk to a counsellor or take medication when they're first diagnosed with depression, so it's vital that a trusted carer or guardian talks to them and explains what depression is. Keeping these lines of communication open mean there's a good chance your child will come and talk to you if they need help.

Ask your child if they can describe what's happening inside. Talk to them about their feelings – do they feel angry or upset?

Tell your child that it's okay for them to talk about anything that may be bothering them if they have to talk to a therapist. Also, explain to your child that going to a therapist isn't a punishment like being sent to the school headteacher; tell them they've not done anything wrong and that the therapist wants to help them find out why they're feeling sad or angry and to help them feel better.

Make sure they understand that it's alright if they want to say things about their family, because you want them to feel better, whatever it takes. Your child and your whole family will come out of the experience happier.

In some therapy sessions, a counsellor may well ask the parents or the child's siblings to take part. This is a good place to sort things out if any of your family members have any concerns about family dynamics.

Explaining a Parent's Depression to a Child

If one of their parents is depressed, a child may not find it easy to understand what's wrong. Explain to them that their parent is trying very hard to get through an illness, and that the depression isn't due to anything they have done wrong. Say that everyone can help the parent get better by being kind and patient, so that your child feels empowered rather than helpless. Use words they will understand to explain what is happening.

You can be a bit more detailed with teenagers, and in both instances give the child lots of opportunities to ask questions.

"I have a strong memory of listening outside a closed door to my mother sobbing and sobbing. In my child's mind, I thought I had done something awful – that I was a terrible person to make my mother cry. She wouldn't come out, she wouldn't talk to me. I must have been around three years old. I felt like I had disappeared. I didn't want to confide in my family, because I thought they'd be disappointed in me.

"Now I understand that it wasn't my fault – but that feeling still haunts me. There was little help or counselling available at that time, so it wasn't until many years later that I realised that my mother had depression. I feel like it would have made a difference in my own life if someone had explained it all to me sooner."

Hatty B.

"With young children, it's best to keep the explanation short but be open to any questions they may ask."

Helping a Child to Understand Suicide

You can't shelter your child or teenager from the grief of bereavement, and you can't shield them from the experience of a relative or friend committing suicide. It's a simple fact of life.

And while it's possible for a child to grasp the idea that their sibling or classmate got very ill and didn't get better, or that their grandmother was very old and had to go to heaven, the idea of someone actually making the decision to kill themselves may be a lot harder for them to come to terms with.

While you should stay open to any questions they may have, if you're talking to a young child it's generally best to keep the explanation short. Try to explain that this person suffered from an illness called depression, which caused them to become very sad. Tell them that they weren't able to think straight because of their illness, and it made them feel like they didn't want to live any more.

With both children and teenagers, you can open a debate about suicide and what the person could have done about getting help and getting well from the depression. Details of the person's suicide may well be requested if you're talking to a teenager. This is just their way of dealing with what has happened in their own minds, and is not simple ghoulish curiosity.

> **"Learning to understand their own sexuality is always an issue during the teenage years, and one fraught with anxiety."**

Explain to your child that feeling sad is normal, especially when there has been a loss or disappointment or when someone is feeling lonely. Make it clear that anyone who feels like life is not worth living can find support and guidance, and make sure your children know that suicide is never the best or only solution, however much it might feel like it is.

Set an example by talking about your own feelings and the positive steps you take to feel better, and tell your children that you are always there to listen if they have problems or sad feelings.

Depression in Teenagers

Depression can sometimes be triggered by hormonal changes, as we have already mentioned. Then there's the pressure, sometimes quite unconscious, from parents who want them to do well at school, mix with the right crowd, get into university or further education, and train for a job. Parents may become so fed up with a teenager's moods that they become critical or angry; or perhaps the parents have troubles of their own and the teen doesn't feel comfortable adding to their burden.

Some teenagers turn to alcohol or drugs because it may be the thing to do in their crowd, or because they see it as a way of coping or even dulling the emotional pain they are experiencing. Teenagers are constantly busy trying to live with the changes taking place in their own bodies, work out where they stand in society, cope with changing relationships, worrying about whether they are smart enough to make it in the world, being concerned as to whether they are one of the cool crowd or disappointed if they're not, and being easily embarrassed and humiliated by others.

Another source of anxiety comes as they learn to understand their own sexuality, which is always an issue during the teenage years. Teenagers have very little life experience to help them keep a perspective, yet they're asked to deal with all of this at once. That's a dangerous time when thoughts of suicide may slip in. Recent studies show that as many as 50% of the teenagers who experience major depression will attempt suicide at least once.

Many teenagers will try to seek a coping mechanism, and they'll find one quickly if they see an example at home of their parents smoking or taking a few drinks to relax when they are stressed.

Whatever the scenario, any number of different triggers are likely to be present that can cause depression to develop and teenagers to feel as though they have nobody to talk to.

You shouldn't ignore the danger signals if you suspect your teenager is depressed, if you think they might have started drinking or taking drugs, if they're exhibiting severe changes in mood, aggressive outbursts, threaten to run away or lock themselves in their rooms. Don't ignore the symptoms: if your teenager won't talk to you, explain that you are concerned about them and persuade – or insist – on a doctor's appointment or a visit to the school guidance counsellor, or teenage suicide helpline.

Adult and teenage depression tends to have similar danger signals.

Let your teenager know that you will always be there to support them, and try to build healthy communication from childhood onwards. It's important that they know that no matter how bad they may be feeling, you are always there to help.

Summing Up

- You may think it's just a phase and will go away, but children do get depressed and parents and carers shouldn't ignore the symptoms.

- In order to rule out any possible underlying physical ailment, the first stop with a child or teenager should always be the family doctor. Usually the family doctor will do a physical check-up first to look for any underlying physical illness, and then discuss the possibility of depression and the various treatments.

- A child with depression may shut themselves away from friends, appear tired and unenthusiastic, and become disinterested in their usual activities.

- Symptoms of depression can also be a warning signal of sexual abuse in some instances.

- You should always seek help from a professional if possible symptoms of depression continue unchanged for more than a week or two.

- Parents should try from earliest childhood to keep the lines of communication open so that their children know they can turn to mum or dad, or another adult relative, to talk about their problems and get an understanding hearing.

- The Internet and television is full of images of war, hunger and violence, and it's difficult to avoid these. It's even more difficult to shelter a child from the difficulties of day-to-day living, the death of a family member, family discord, playground bullying or parental divorce, the loss of a much-loved pet, moving to a new neighbourhood or losing a best friend.

- It is important not to just ignore these warning signs in a child, or put them down to teenage moods or growing pains.

- Triggers may include the loss of a loved person or pet, moving house, changing school, family discord or parental separation/divorce, being bullied or having difficulty with a teacher.

- Younger children may show depression by becoming withdrawn and moody, failing in school, becoming disruptive, given to temper tantrums or even hitting and biting.

- Because of the possible serious ramifications of depression in children, it's probably better to err on the side of caution and seek professional help.

7

Health Problems Connected to Depression

I t's easy to see that a person suffering a serious illness would feel depressed about their situation, but did you know that there is a link between depression and the onset of some medical conditions? Either as a result or a contributing factor, depression is a component of a number of other diseases.

Depression and Obesity – The Catch 22 Situation

"While it's true that some overweight people may become depressed because they hate the way they look, or feel they are socially isolated due to their weight, studies seem to show that in a high percentage of cases, the depression comes first, not as a result of being overweight."

While it may not be the one that springs to mind at first, recent studies show that there is a link between depression and obesity. Much of the current research centres on something called the HPA axis, a hormonal pathway in the brain which is linked to obesity, behavioural problems, and depression in children. In other words, if you're depressed, you may be more likely to be overweight.

It seems that rather than being a result of being overweight, in a high percentage of cases the depression actually comes first. (That said, some overweight people do also become depressed because they are made to feel bad about the way they look, or feel that they are socially isolated due to their weight). Obese adults appear often to have been depressed as children and/or adolescents, according to some studies.

Depression is believed to be caused by low serotonin levels, and one theory is that someone who is depressed may take to eating larger amounts than normal in a subconscious attempt to boost these levels. Unfortunately, this is more likely to lead to the weight gain observed in some depressed patients, and therefore to a downward spiral of depression and overeating.

This means that without realising it, they may be trying to cure their depression with food but are actually adding to their problems as additional health risks come with being seriously overweight. If you are depressed and overweight, this may be something to talk over with your doctor.

The need to overeat could potentially be removed if the person's serotonin uptake is more effective. Fortunately, this is potentially possible and researchers are currently looking into the effects of antidepressant SSRIs for this reason.

The Impact of Stress on Your Mood

As anyone suffering from trauma-triggered stress will already appreciate, research from the Mayo Clinic has found that chronic stress can create depression. For some people, a seemingly stressful situation will roll off like water off a duck's back, while for others the situation will trigger major anxiety. Also, some of us can learn from our parents and older relatives ways of coping that allow us to keep stress in perspective.

Everyone has their own way of responding to stress and there doesn't seem to be any decisive reason for this. People seem to simply have varying levels of vulnerability to stress.

Stress can be alleviated by taking care of yourself – eat nutritious food, get some exercise every day or as often as you can, make sure you get enough sleep and avoid using alcohol or other addictive substances. Better to deal with problems than try to drown them. Some people find it really helpful to practice relaxation techniques like yoga, massage, meditation and deep breathing – as these help with depression.

Rather than clearing it up, things like smoking, illegal drugs and alcohol only mask stress in the short-term. It's well known that some people turn to drink or drugs as a means of alleviating stress, but this is a learned behaviour that doesn't really help.

Depression and Eating Disorders

Eating disorders only seem to have been recognised in relatively recent years. It is unclear whether this is because anorexia and bulimia are increasing at a rate that has made them recognised as illnesses in themselves, or whether it is because they are a relatively new phenomenon.

Anorexics starve themselves voluntarily to the point of emaciation, and will find all sorts of excuses to avoid situations involving food, including family meal times. Using laxatives or vomiting to purge after eating a large amount of food in a binge is the primary symptom of bulimia. The starvation and lack of nutrition can lead to serious health complications and even death, and sufferers need medical intervention as soon as possible.

Despite sometimes massive weight loss, sufferers of both conditions still consider themselves to be "fat". Talk to your doctor if you fear you or someone you care about is engaged in these practices.

Certainly, in times when there wasn't such an abundance of food, there was probably little problem with overeating and purging through vomiting or laxatives among working people. The growth of eating disorders is likely to be at least in part down to modern day pressures to have a model-thin appearance, though it's probable that there has always been some manifestation of eating disorders.

Whether the depression follows the emotional problems and physical deprivation of the eating disorder, or whether the eating disorder arises from the depression, is still a subject for lively debate. There is a sort of chicken-and-egg relationship between certain eating disorders and depression, and it's also known that some depressed people may overeat in an unconscious bid to raise their serotonin levels and in turn elevate their mood.

Depression and eating disorders – including overeating, compulsive eating, bulimia and anorexia – can sometimes be linked, and it's important to be aware of this risk.

Depression and Addiction

Many alcoholics who try to quit drinking find it hard because depression usually sets in when they first withdraw from alcohol, making the craving for a drink 'to take off the edge' much stronger and harder to resist. It is believed that 30-50% of alcoholics also suffer from depression. Alcoholism and depression have a number of symptoms in common, though no studies so far have shown that alcoholism actually causes depression.

People coping with a personal trauma or trying to control sadness or other emotional pain will often drink to excess. As we discuss in The Essential Guide to Alcoholism, although alcohol makes you feel better when you first have a drink or two, the good mood doesn't last because alcohol can actually spark depressed feelings in the let-down which follows the alcohol high.

Alcohol has the effect of impairing your judgement while increasing the likelihood of impetuous or reckless behaviour. Alcoholics are also known for drug overdoses. Your risk of suicide can also be increased if you are depressed and start drinking heavily, as the alcohol intensifies your suicidal thoughts and lessens your inhibitions. Attempts to commit suicide by deliberately driving recklessly are common, or accidental death may occur as a result of driving while impaired by alcohol or drugs.

If you, or a friend, are depressed and drinking heavily, it is important that you seek medical attention because of the heightened suicide risks.

Symptoms Linking Alcoholism and Depression

- Your risk of developing alcoholism or depression is higher if either health problem is an issue in your family.

- Drinking alcohol may cause a relapse in your condition if you are recovering from a depressive episode.

- Over the space of three or four weeks drinking alcohol can appear to reduce the symptoms of depression, however when the alcohol intake stops those symptoms will return even stronger.

- If you are an alcoholic with a history of depression, you should talk to your doctor or healthcare professional about close monitoring when you are in the early stages of withdrawal.

- Alcohol can intensify the feeling of depression.

Less Common Conditions

Huntingdon's Disease

An abnormal gene causes Huntingdon's disease, a condition you inherit from your parents. Depression, mood swings and irritability are among the early warning symptoms of Huntingdon's disease, along with perceptual problems that lead to difficulties driving and learning new things, and a deterioration in memory and decision-making skills.

Emotional disturbance, uncontrolled movements and loss of intellectual faculties are among the symptoms of this condition.

Depression and Schizophrenia

Someone's level of suffering from schizophrenia can be increased if they experience depression as well – which is very common. It is not fully understood why the two illnesses occur together but it's probably not coincidental. As you can see, the co-relation of depression and schizophrenia is a complex and tangled one.

Sometimes the medications used to treat schizophrenic symptoms may also lead to depression as a side effect. Suicide attempts are also more likely if the person also has depression. Schizophrenia's uncontrolled moods are possibly the cause of depression in some cases. Depression may occur as a result of the physical neglect that is often part of the lifestyle of someone with schizophrenia, as this can result in the person becoming physically run-down.

Depression can sometimes be triggered by alcohol and recreational drugs, and some people with schizophrenia will use these to relieve their symptoms.

Before setting a course of treatment, when a doctor considers the onset of depression in a patient diagnosed with schizophrenia, they will look at lifestyle, physical health, medications and other factors for this reason.

Anxiety Conditions and Depression

According to a 2005 survey, about 58% of people diagnosed with depression also suffered from some form of anxiety. While they may worry, like the rest of us perhaps, about work, money, and their families, they also get overly anxious about relatively minor matters such as being organised, keeping their homes tidy and having projects finished on time.

Hypochondria, OCD, post traumatic stress disorder, social phobia and separation anxiety are just some of the phobias and anxiety disorders out there. GAD (generalised anxiety disorder) is a catch-all title for serious anxiety difficulties that don't result from other individual anxiety disorders, such as separation anxiety or social phobia, each of which stem from a specific fear.

These conditions will affect everyone differently – for instance, fewer men suffer from generalised anxiety disorder (GAD) than women. The day-to-day lives of people with GAD will be made much more difficult by the uncontrollable anxiety they feel about everyday events. Other mental issues tend to be a much better problem for young people with GAD than those in the general population, as they will often fail to reach their full potential in school and their early careers. These young people are also more likely to get involved with substance abuse.

Generalised Anxiety Disorder – The Symptoms

The following are some signs that you may be experiencing generalised anxiety disorder:

- You'll often feel anxious about something for months on end, and get extremely worried or stressed out about relatively ordinary events, such as a school test or work review.

- Your relationships, friendships and work are suffering as a result of your anxiety.

- You often get tired out.

- You have disturbing dreams, sleep restlessly, or struggle to sleep at all.

- Your muscles are tense and you have difficulty concentrating.

- You feel restless and tense most of the time.

- You can't control the amount of worrying you do, and you worry excessively, sometimes about relatively minor things.

Only your health care professional can offer you a proper diagnosis after consideration of symptoms, background, lifestyle and a physical check-up. Talk to your doctor or a counsellor for help. As usual, this list should not be used to diagnose yourself or anyone else with GAD.

You can learn to keep a balanced perception of events through counselling and therapy, and anxiety disorders are treatable if you're able to relearn your thinking into positive, rather than negative thoughts. Medications are also necessary in some cases.

Psychotic Depression

Paranoid tendencies, seeing things that aren't there, hearing voices and erratic behaviours all characterise this extreme form of depression. Although this may sound quite similar to the symptoms of schizophrenia, they are different in that people with psychotic depression are usually very aware that words whispered in their ears may come from voices that don't exist and the things they see may not actually be real.

This rather frightening sounding type of depression is not particularly rare: approximately 25% of people who are admitted to hospital because of depression are suffering from the symptoms of psychotic depression. Many people with this condition will attempt to hide it because they realise that these things are not real, and because they realise that talking about them may make them sound "crazy".

This not only makes it hard to diagnose, but means that the symptoms may worsen to a point where they can no longer be hidden before they are noticed by other people, meaning that the person goes untreated for too long a time. It can be a great source of shame. Suicide risk in those with this condition is quite high as a result, as is the risk of bipolar depression and relapses of psychotic depression.

Factors contributing to the development of this illness according to recent research include family history, hormonal imbalances and previous bipolar depression, but the exact cause of the condition is not yet known. Because childbirth results in a fluctuation of hormones (see Chapter One), the hormone imbalance factor can lead to psychotic depression being an offshoot of postnatal depression.

Characteristics of psychotic depression can include:

- Intense distress and worry.
- Seeing things.
- Other anxiety disorders.

- Symptoms of paranoia and hypochondria.
- Delusions and the sense of not being able to control your own thoughts.
- Disturbed sleep, often with frightening nightmares.

Depression and Health Anxiety

One anxiety disorder you're likely to have heard of is health anxiety, which is also known as hypochondria or hypochondriasis. Seeing every muscle twitch or cough as a potential symptom of any number of different illnesses, people with this condition can become obsessed with their own physical state. They constantly seek reassurance that they're not seriously ill, while at the same time coming up with new symptoms to counter any arguments that they are well.

Such worry about physical illness can trigger anxiety attacks. Sadly, there's an old saying, 'just because you're paranoid doesn't mean to say they aren't after you', and this can be applied to hypochondria, too. Friends, family and sometimes even doctors can become impatient with them, as they can be very difficult to convince that they are in good health.

But in some cases, a genuine illness could be ignored in everyone's eagerness to disregard the symptoms someone with hypochondria is claiming to have.

Someone with this condition can quickly find that their relationship with medical professionals and other people in their life is becoming strained, and the symptoms of this condition can really prevent them from enjoying an ordinary life.

Health anxiety can manifest through the following symptoms, among others:

- A strong belief that the individual is suffering from a serious disease.
- Suspicion of any healthy diagnosis received from a doctor.
- Misinterpreting and diagnosing one's own symptoms.
- Complaints of numerous vague aches and pains that change over short periods of time.
- Constant checking out oneself for physical changes that might indicate illness.
- Fear of dying through illness.

Hypochondria can be triggered in some cases by the long illness or death of a loved one or friend, by increased personal stress, by a very real fear of an illness which grows out of proportion, and by ill health in childhood. A lack of motivation, depression, panic attacks, loss of appetite, no interest in sex, loss of interest in social life or other activities and self-consciousness are among the serious consequences that can occur as a result of this condition.

All the while, any number of different humour columnists will continue to make jokes about hypochondria.

Antidepressant medications, hypnotherapy and cognitive behavioural therapy have all been used to successfully treat this condition.

Post Traumatic Stress Disorder

It is accepted now that for many people the experience and the trauma of war, of being fired upon, being injured, or seeing friends injured or killed, can trigger PTSD. It is described as 'a normal reaction to an abnormal situation, a deeply shocking or disturbing experience' by Harley Street stress consultant David Reeves in an article on PTSD published on the Mindtech Association web site.

"Serious psychiatric problems" meant that around 1.5% of military personnel had to be evacuated from Iraq home to Britain in 2006, according to the Ministry of Defence. In the decade since then, the Ministry of Defence have reported that the rates of diagnosed mental health conditions in serving Armed Forces personnel have doubled to around 3% (which is still slightly lower than the rate in the general public, 4–5% of whom suffer from PTSD).

Experts believe that the figure may actually be considerably higher, but that some soldiers are reluctant to admit to having problems, such as flashbacks of painful memories, feelings of isolation or loss of control, etc, because they are either ashamed or they are afraid that being diagnosed with PTSD will affect their military careers.

In the US, the number of veterans with PTSD varies depending on where they served: Around 11-20% of those who served in Iraq, 12% of those who served in the Gulf War and up to 30% of those who served in Vietnam.

Thousands of British troops may have been diagnosed with PTSD. As a result of the suffering of soldiers returning from various wars and "peacekeeping missions", PTSD, or post-traumatic stress disorder, is something that has been brought to public attention a great deal in recent years. There is some evidence to suggest that many young men were executed during the First World War for being deserters and cowards, when in fact they were simply unable to control their behaviour due to this mental illness.

A sense of helplessness, terror and intense fear as a result of a sudden life threatening event will often be the cause of PTSD – things like being under fire during war, experiencing a sexual assault or ongoing sexual abuse, or a severe car accident. For a diagnosis of PTSD the symptoms usually are expected to be present for longer than three months.

Violent outbursts due to disorientation are a symptom of the disorder, as are difficulty sleeping, anxiety attacks, difficulty concentrating, flashbacks and loss of control.

PTSD usually results from the experience of a life threatening trauma, or one that is perceived as life threatening. The effects can be reduced by intervention as soon as feasible after the traumatic event, called structured stress debriefings, to help the person cope and come to terms with the experience. Alcohol/drug abuse, depression, GAD, panic disorder or another identifiable mental health component are also present in about 80% of people diagnosed with PTSD.

The recent trauma is generally used as a key factor in diagnosing the condition, as its similarities with depression and anxiety disorders can make it very difficult to diagnose.

Treatment usually involves antidepressant drugs, psychotherapy and counselling, and education to help the patient understand what is happening. It's important to treat all conditions simultaneously because of the number of disorders than can coexist with PTSD.

Summing Up

- It's not always clear whether depression has occurred as a result of a coexisting illness, or if the other illness has occurred because of the depression. This is sometimes described as a chicken-and-egg relationship (as in "which came first?")

- PTSD can easily be triggered by the stress of a battle situation, where military personnel have their lives in jeopardy, see friends killed or maimed, or are forced to take the life of another human being.

- There are a number of mental illnesses that contain a depressive element, and some that lead to depression and vice versa.

- Underlying physical ailments could be to blame for certain depressive symptoms, so anyone who thinks they may have depression should be sure to visit their GP for a physical check-up.

- The reason that depression plays a major or minor role in many other health issues will likely be made clear by future discoveries. All we know for now is that the links do exist.

- We can understand that someone with a serious medical condition may feel depressed about their circumstances, and a survivor of war, natural disaster or major car crash might well feel depressed for some time afterwards as they recover. Likewise, depression stemming from stress or as part of general anxiety disorder is easy to understand, but it's harder to grasp the connection between eating disorders or hypochondria and depression.

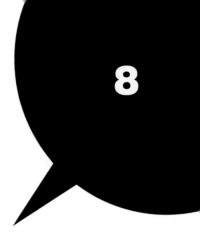

8

Looking Forward: Life with Depression

t's hard to look ahead when you're struggling to just get through the next hour, the next day. The future may seem like a strange concept when you're deep in a depressive episode. But your life will go on: your depression will get easier to deal with, and there will come a day when you feel like yourself again. You may even feel like you've missed out while you were getting through that depressive episode, and feel an imperative to get extra fulfilment from your work and personal life.

But what if you get depressed again? It's a scary thought to consider.

"I was free to get on with my life. The things that had haunted me from childhood had been a burden, and I'd finally dropped it. But life seemed to get on top of me again when I stopped seeing my therapist and no longer had his support to rely on. I was depressed again. I couldn't cope with life, and it made me feel so weak. Is there anything I can do to help myself?

"Lurching from one depression to another is no fun. My counsellor was able to pull me out of it, this time, but how many more times would it happen?"

Paul M.

The Future

Statistics show that one in three people who have had depression will experience another episode within a year; 50-80% will have another episode of depression within their lifetime.

Sometimes the reason for a relapse is simple: either the patient was not on a long enough course of antidepressants, or the failure to include psychotherapy counselling led to serious unresolved issues triggering further depressions. Sometimes people start to feel better and decide to quit with the medication before it has run its course – and this can lead to a further episode of depression.

Many people experience a recurrence of depression, though a lucky few may not. As they grow older, some people will experience more frequent and longer bouts of depression.

Making Things Better

Don't feel helpless – you are empowered because you have things that you can do to recover from this depression. Accepting that you can survive another episode of depression if you've already survived your first is a big step forward in accepting your condition. It won't be fun, but you now know what to expect and you know to seek help.

You need to recognise that relapses do occur, and if it happens to you then it's not your fault. All you can do is do what you can to get through it. It's very important that you don't beat yourself up or play the blame game if you do get depressed – recognise that you've done everything you could to avoid this.

The Easy Stuff

Always follow your doctor's orders: if you're put on antidepressants, make sure you take them exactly as prescribed and don't stop until you're told to. Many counsellors will suggest going on a maintenance program rather than quitting counselling 'cold turkey'.

If your bad feelings could be triggered by personal issues, consider talking to a therapist to work on your depression. This allows you to discuss any further anxieties that come up over time even though you are feeling better, and the support the counsellor is able to give helps you remain well.

If you feel your counselling has run its course and are ready to stop altogether, it's generally best to reduce the frequency of your visits rather than stopping suddenly. This gives you time to venture out into the world and see if your depression is truly at bay, while you know you still have the support of your counsellor just a telephone call away. But if you stop counselling before you're really ready, you may be throwing away the regular support that your counsellor provides and this could lead to slipping back into depression.

Over time, you will learn to control your triggers and your counsellor can help by encouraging you to identify the triggers that may cause you to feel depressed. Some of these are triggers that you can control; others are triggers that are beyond your control.

The Tricky Bits

You will probably notice that there are some warning signs that you are becoming depressed; perhaps you are more tired than usual, lethargic, and less interested in things you normally enjoy. This is where you should remember the effects of positive thinking, of overlaying negative thoughts about yourself and your situation with positive ones.

If you need help from your therapist or doctor, do not hesitate to contact them. There are things that you can do to help yourself, though. The best thing you can do for yourself is to stay vigilant: If your hopes for the future are becoming dimmed or your thoughts and view of the world are becoming negative, be aware that this could be a sign of another depressive episode.

Get together with upbeat people for a relaxing chat or an outing. Consider taking a holiday or even a day trip somewhere you want to visit. Your doctor or counsellor should have taught you some relaxation and breathing exercises already – use these. These are all things that should lift your mood, and should be part of your daily regimen, your own Plan A for avoiding depression.

Try and revitalise your day with a new perspective or a change of scene. These should be social activities as well as some of the solitary hobbies you may like. Make sure you are getting out and about for activities in the fresh air and sunshine, eat plenty of fresh fruit and vegetables and note your alcohol and caffeine intake.

Your depression may well have been sparked by a recognisable trigger. Try not to feel bad if something you can't control gets you down – learn to accept and understand your condition.

Triggers You Can Control

Some of these triggers can be avoided, or even resolved:

- Unhealthy diet.
- Arguments with loved ones.
- Being unhappy at work, or being stressed or overworked.
- Lack of "me" time or time off.
- Drinking alcohol, smoking or the use of illegal drugs.
- Long commuting times.
- Being bullied at work.
- Not getting enough exercise, sleep and relaxation.

Learn to eat a well-balanced diet, avoid alcohol, exercise regularly, and make sure you get enough sleep. You can do something about all or most of the potential triggers in the list above. Be sure to remember to get out and do things that you enjoy, and do your relaxation exercises as often as you can.

If there's always a fight at a get-together, try to talk to the people involved beforehand and settle the matter – or else politely decline the invitation and give your reasons. Identify the causes and source of any family conflicts and try to deal with it accordingly.

You'd be surprised how many adults report that they are bullied at work, and the result can be lost work time, depression and even suicide. Bullying at work can be a real issue. Bullying at work requires an effective workplace policy, and according to the Andrea Adams Trust, a non-profit charity focussing on bullying in the workplace, at least 40% of UK organisations don't have this. According to a survey published by TUC in 2015, managers are responsible for 72% of all instances of workplace bullying.

Every year 18.9 million working days are lost to industry as a direct result of workplace bullying, costing the UK economy 6 billion pounds and massively impacting on productivity, creativity, morale and general employee wellbeing. At some point during their working lives, it is believed that at least 25% of people will be bullied.

If your job is triggering depression, take action:

- **Inform your manager or supervisor** – or go higher if they are the ones doing the bullying. HR can be invaluable in these cases. Request a conflict negotiation. If you have a union representative, talk to them. Talk to a lawyer if nothing else works. Depression is serious and you have to do what it takes to avoid suffering from repeated episodes. It may be necessary to look for a new job or move to a new location – though this can be difficult in the current economic climate.

- **Struggling with the commute?** Moving to a house nearer to your work or a job nearer your home isn't always an option, but there are still things you can do to make your commute more enjoyable. See what you can do to make the travel time more productive or enjoyable – try taking along a good book, listening to some music or writing something.

- **Cut out any recreational drugs, alcohol and smoking.** If you aren't able to quit by yourself, ask at your local wellness clinic or doctor's surgery about local smoking/drinking/drug addiction programmes, or seek help from your doctor. If there's no group near you – and your local health unit or doctor's office should know – then consider starting your own.

- **Take control of the things you can control.**

- **Take any holidays that are owed to you and use them.** Do something you enjoy – it doesn't have to cost the earth. Doing something relaxing, preferably in a change of scenery, can be quite a refreshing boost.

- **The same holds true if you are overworked or unhappy in your job.** Talk to the higher ups and your co-workers to see what can be done to redistribute the workload or make the general work ambience more pleasant and more interesting.

Some Triggers Are Harder to Control

If the following events occur, you may need to seek support and guidance in coping as they are stressful and potential triggers for depression.

- Death of a loved one.

- Losing your job.

- Problems with money.

- Starting in a new job.

- Moving house.

- Accidents.

- Serious illness (your own or that of a loved one).

- Divorce.

When dealing with one of these, it's helpful to sit down and list the problems, how you feel, and what you can actually do about it. It may help to have a loved one or close friend sit down with you to discuss the problems and how you can cope. Some of these triggers won't even give you any warning before they occur, and all you can do is learn to understand that some events and situations cannot be avoided.

Another survival method suggested by therapists is to keep a journal in which you write down your feelings and the associated events each day. If you need to develop a sense of being in control, writing a to-do list can be a great way to cope with these issues. Consider having a Plan A and a Plan B. Plan B is for those days when you simply don't want to get out of bed in the morning, the days when depression creeps up and you don't care what happens.

Try to see this as an opportunity to get a new perspective on your life, or to develop a mutually supportive relationship with a loved one. Working on these problems with someone you trust can really help the two of you to grow closer.

Many people report feeling lighter after writing down the things that have been bothering them. If you need a way of getting your thoughts and feelings in order, a journal is a great way to keep a record of events and compare them against your mood. It doesn't need to be a great literary work – see it as a form of therapy. Be sure to keep the journal in a safe place or destroy any pages you don't want others to read, as if your writing contains any angry or derogatory remarks about your nearest and dearest this can easily spark a conflict which will do nothing to improve your mood! You don't want to accidentally ruin an otherwise healthy relationship by allowing the target of your ill feelings to accidentally read about it.

Figure out a daily routine that allows you to recognise possible triggers and act to minimise their impact, while keeping to a good diet and exercise plan.

But the moment you feel that you really are becoming depressed, get help. Come up with a second plan that will get you moving on days when you're feeling depressed, as this is when you most need a support system: a friend you can call who'll drop by to visit or meet you out for a coffee or a walk and a chat, or a supportive therapy group with other people who experience depression.

Borderline depressed days can really be made easier through a buddy system, and you'll be surprised how many people will be on board to help.

What You Can Do if Your Friend Is Depressed

1   Remember that your friend didn't choose to have depression, and be patient with them.

2   Send them a card, a text or an email – maintain a communication link. Isolation may seem appealing to them, but it won't help so don't let them fall into that trap. Your friend needs you most when they're depressed, even if they aren't the best company right now.

3   Find out what services are available locally, and provide moral support by offering to go along to any meetings with them.

4   Be aware of any mood changes or worsening of the depression, and encourage your friend or loved one to go to the doctor or contact a health professional.

5   Be encouraging, find something about them to praise and bite back any criticisms.

6   Talk to them about what's going on, or be prepared to be silent and listen.

When Should You Stop the Medication or Counselling?

Always take your pills as directed – antidepressants usually take weeks to show their effectiveness, so be patient. Always take medication as your doctor advises, and always consult them before you stop taking it. Some people might start feeling much better very quickly and stop taking their medication because they think they're already cured. It's important to remember that just because you're feeling better, it doesn't mean the job is done.

Never stop taking your medication without checking with your doctor first – it takes time to get those brain chemicals back in balance.

The same rule applies to therapy, even if you're feeling good and feel that you've got a handle on the issues that triggered your depression. Either way, stopping cold turkey in your counselling can be as bad as stopping cold turkey with medication.

Certain therapists will prefer to work slowly, while others recommend a short, intensive series of visits. Whichever approach they prefer, most will recommend a gradual weaning away from your regular visits and encourage you to come to maintenance appointments that will slowly become less frequent before tailing off completely.

Helping Yourself

1 Give yourself time to get back on form: Don't have unfeasibly high expectations for yourself just because you're feeling better.

2 Ask your co-workers, relatives and friends for their support and assistance.

3 Be sure to hang out with friends as well as on your own. Take care of yourself by getting all the sleep you need, eating well and exercising.

4 Think positively; try to overlay negative thoughts with positive ones.

5 Set up support systems so you always have a reason to get out of bed in the morning and there's an understanding friend or a therapy group buddy that you can talk to.

6 When faced with a big project or a major depression trigger, try to list the step-by-step actions you need to take, so that you feel in control.

7 Finally, know when you need to seek outside help and support from your medical doctor or your counsellor.

Are there things you do that make you feel better? This list is just a short suggestion – there are bound to be plenty more antidepressant standbys that you can add.

Summing Up

- There's a very real risk of relapse for anyone who has experienced an episode of depression in the past.

- Set about staving off further episodes by coming up with an action plan. Set up your support system and resources so that when you feel that dull sense of depression creeping in, you're ready to man the barricades.

- Try to deal with personal differences before the event if you have a family event coming up that you know will involve some sort of argument. When you're dealing with depression triggers like this, learn when you can avoid them or what you can do to resolve or control the problem.

- For people in a relationship with someone with depression, this could be an opportunity for the two of you to renew your relationship on a stronger footing and a chance to develop a closer lifestyle by working together to identify and resolve depression triggers.

- Given the bad effects of depression and the way everything, especially decision making and planning, can become too much bother, it's a good idea to think of contingency plans before you become depressed again.

Help List

Emergency Helplines

If you are suicidal or experiencing a crisis, you can call these numbers to speak to a counsellor. If you'd rather, you could also travel to your nearest hospital's emergency room and tell a nurse or doctor there what's happening.

APNI – Association for Post-Natal Illness

Apni.org
Address: 145 Dawes Road, Fulham, London, SW6 7EB
Tel: 0207 386 0868
Email: info@apni.org
APNI offers support for those suffering from postnatal illnesses such as postnatal depression. They also encourage research and aim to raise public awareness of the illness. You can contact them by telephone or email. The Samaritans or Family Lives (0808 800 2222) can be contacted if you need urgent help outside of office hours.

Childline

www.childline.org.uk
Address: NSPCC, Weston House, 42 Curtain Road, London, EC2A 3NH
Tel: 0800 1111 (helpline for children)
Email: Contact form on website (https://www.childline.org.uk/get-support/ask-sam/ask-sam-a-question/)
If you're a child or young person in the UK, you can call Childline to talk about your problems for free. Children 1st provide this service in Scotland, and NSPCC in England. Any problem can be discussed on this confidential service including running away from home, bullying, gangs, drugs, depression, pregnancy and abuse.

Crime Victims Helpline (Ireland)

https://crimevictimshelpline.ie
Tel: Freephone 116 006
Email: Info@crimevictimshelpline.ie
Witnesses and victims of crime in the Republic of Ireland can contact this helpline for support. Victim Support provide a similar service in the UK.

Family Lives (Parentline Plus)

https://www.familylives.org.uk

Address: 15-17 The Broadway, Hatfield, Hertfordshire, AL9 5HZ

Tel: 0808 800 2222 (helpline)

Email: askus@familylives.org.uk

A national charity that works for parents, with parents. The organisation offers training, support groups, workshops and local services as well as a great helpline. There's also plenty of great information on their website.

National Drugs Helpline

www.talktofrank.com

Tel: 0300 123 6600

Email: frank@talktofrank.com

A free, confidential helpline for people addicted to drugs and their families, open 24/7.

The Samaritans UK

www.samaritans.org

Address: Chris, PO Box 9090, Stirling, FK8 2SA

Tel: 084 57 909090 (helpline) / 1850 609090 (helpline Ireland)

Email: jo@samaritans.org

Samaritans provides a confidential support service for people who are depressed, feeling distressed or considering suicide. The service is available 24 hours a day in the UK and Ireland.

Victim Support

www.victimsupport.org.uk

Find your nearest Victim Support office at www.victimsupport.org.uk/help-and-support/get-help/support-near-you

Tel: 08 08 16 89 (Supportline)

Email: Contact form on website.

Victim Support provide help to victims of crime in the UK. They have offices across the UK, and you can find your local office through their website. If you need help outside of office hours, call the Samaritans instead. See Crime Victims Helpline for support in the Republic of Ireland.

Women's Aid

www.womensaid.org.uk

Address: Women's Aid Federation of England, PO BOX 3245, Bristol BS2 2EH

Tel: 0808 2000 247 (Helpline)

Email: Helpline@womensaid.org.uk

Women's Aid provide information and support for women experiencing sexual abuse or domestic violence, and a 24-hour national helpline on domestic violence.

Youthline

www.youthlineuk.com

Address: The Lodge, Coopers Hill, Bagshot Road, Bracknell, Berkshire, RG12 7QS

Tel: 01344 311200

Email: ask@youthlineuk.com

Youthline provides free, confidential counselling in Berkshire to children aged 8-11 and their families, and to young people about anything from drugs to bullying.

Resources

If you need information about organisations that help with depression and some of its attendant problems, check out the list below.

Action on Addiction

www.actiononaddiction.org.uk

Address: East Knoyle, Wiltshire, SP3 6BE

Tel: 0845 1264130 (helpline)

Charity to help all those affected by addictions, including research and family support.

Addaction

www.addaction.org.uk

Address: Part Lower Ground Floor, Gate House, 1-3 St. John's Square, London EC1m 4DH

Tel: 020 7251 5860

Email: Webchat on site (https://www.addaction.org.uk/webchat)

Addaction's website provides help and guidance for people addicted to drugs or alcohol.

Al-Anon UK

www.al-anonuk.org.uk

Helpline: 0800 0086 811 / 01 873 2699 (EIRE)

General Service Office

Address: Al-Anon Family Groups, 57 Great Suffolk Street, London SE1 0BB

Tel: 020 7593 2070

Contact form: https://www.al-anonuk.org.uk/send-an-email/

Republic of Ireland

Address: Al-Anon Information Centre, Room 5, 5 Capel Street, Dublin 1, EIRE

Tel: 01 878 3624

Email: info@alanon.ie

Website: alanon.ie

Northern Ireland

Address: Al-Anon, Peace House, 224 Lisburn Road, Belfast BT9 6GE
Tel: 02890 68 2368
Email: See General Service contact form.
Al-Anon offer meetings and support groups aimed at the families and friends of alcoholics and people trying to give up drinking.

Alcoholics Anonymous

www.alcoholics-anonymous.org.uk
Address: PO Box 1, 10 Toft Green, York, YO1 7ND
Tel: 0800 9177 650 (helpline)
Email: help@aamail.org
Organises support groups and meetings for people trying to give up drinking alcohol. Alcoholics Anonymous does not charge fees or have religious or political affiliations. AA is a support organisation that help people all over the world with their alcohol addictions. You can find a group near you or learn more about the organisation by checking out the website.

Alcoholics Anonymous Ireland

http://www.alcoholicsanonymous.ie
Address: Unit 2, Block C, Santry Business Park, Swords Road, Dublin 9, EIRE
Tel: 353 18420700
Email: Gso@alcoholicsanonymous.ie
"Our primary purpose is to stay sober and help other alcoholics to achieve sobriety." The Republic of Ireland's Alcoholics Anonymous group.

Association for the Study of Obesity

www.aso.org.uk
Address: ASO, PO Box 5413, Brighton BN50 8HH
Tel: 07847 2438309 (Office Hours: Tuesday to Thursday, 9.30am to 2.30pm)
Email: ASOoffice@aso.org.uk
Dedicated to the understanding and treatment of obesity, this organisation was first set up in 1967. Although the site is not aimed at parents, there is good advice, useful links and contacts. They aim to spread awareness of obesity and the impacts it can have on a person's health, as well as promote the prevention and treatment of the condition and research and understand its causes. The site also has some handy videos and information to use in the classroom.

Bipolar Aware
Bipolaraware.co.uk

Email: Info@bipolaraware.co.uk

A 'family guide' to bipolar disorder, this self-help web site containing information about diagnosis, treatments, education, etc. It also has forums and anecdotal material. The site was established by Mark Hannant to help others with this illness. Mr Hannant states he is not a medical or mental health professional.

The Black Dog
www.theblackdog.net

An Irish website aimed at men with mental and psychological health issues. It features an on-site email form, chatrooms, discussion groups and links to other resources.

Combat Stress
www.combatstress.org.uk

Address: Tyrwhitt House, Oaklawn Road, Leatherhead, Surrey, KT22 0BX

Tel: 0800 138 1619 (Helpline)

Email: helpline@combatstress.org.uk

Combat Stress have a regional network of welfare officers available to visit discharged members of the military and merchant navy at home or in hospital. They aim to support them through any metal health issues, including PTSD.

Dublin Rape Crisis Centre
www.drcc.ie

Address: 70 Lower Leeson Street, Dublin 2, Republic of Ireland

Tel: 1800 778888 (freephone)

Email: rrc@indigo.ie

Provides contact details, help and resources for victims of rape and other sex crimes. Lists contact details for centres around Ireland. Has a 24 hour a day freephone hotline.

Freedom from Torture (Medical Foundation for the Care of Victims of Torture)
https://www.freedomfromtorture.org

Address: Medical Foundation London, 111 Isledon Road, Islington, London, N7 7JW

Tel: 020 7697 7777

Contact form: https://www.freedomfromtorture.org/contact-us

Site has news, facts, and survivor stories as well as a treatment referral facility. Also email form on website. Freedom from Torture provide specialist psychological therapy to help asylum seekers and refugees who have survived torture to recover and rebuild their lives in the UK. They also provide training for professionals working with torture survivors.

GROW

www.grow.ie
Tel: 1890 474474 (infoline)
Email: info@grow.ie
An Irish support group of people who suffer or have suffered from mental illness. Local groups in many areas. Grow is a mental health organisation supporting people who have suffered or are suffering from mental health problems. Has a '12-step' programme.

Health.com

http://www.health.com/depression
Those experiencing depression (and those living with them) may find some helpful information on health.com, which has articles about many different conditions.

Inspire

https://www.inspirewellbeing.org
Address: Inspire, Lombard House, 10-20 Lombard Street, Belfast BT1 1RD
Tel: 028 9032 8474
Email: hello@inspirewellbeing.org
Support services across Northern Ireland includes housing schemes, home support, advocacy and research as well as public education and information. Inspire offers a range of services that provide support in the areas of mental health and learning disability, across a range of areas.

Internet Mental Health

www.mentalhealth.com
A free online encyclopedia with information about a load of different mental health conditions.

Just Fight On! (Workplace Bullying Support Group Network)

www.jfo.org.uk/
Tel: 08457 47 47 47
Email: jo@jfo.org.uk
Contact information, including website and email addresses, is available under each member group's link. A not-for-profit anti-bullying organisation.

Kidscape

www.kidscape.org.uk

Address: 2 Grosvenor Gardens, London, SW1W 0DH

Tel: 020 7730 3300 (helpline)

Email: info@kidscape.org.uk

Kidscape believes that protecting children from harm is key, and advises children experiencing bullying to contact Childline (see above). Kidscape's mission is to provide children, families, carers and professionals with advice, training and practical tools to prevent bullying and protect young lives. They provide professionals, children and families with information and guidance to keep kids safe. Their website has loads of great resources and helpful contacts.

MedicineNet

www.medicinenet.com

An American website with lots of great information about depression and similar conditions.

Mind

www.mind.org.uk

Address: 15–19 Broadway, London, E15 4BQ

Wales: 3rd Floor, Castlebridge 4, Castlebridge, 5-19 Cowbridge Road East, Cardiff CF11 9AB

Tel: 0300 123 3393 (infoline)

Email: info@mind.org.uk

Mind provides advice and support to empower anyone experiencing a mental health problem.

Narcotics Anonymous Ireland

www.na-ireland.org

Address: PO Box 13033, 14b Upper Kevin Street, Dublin 8

Tel: +353 (0)1-6728000 (information line)

Email: info@na-ireland.org

Helpline numbers for four areas and online email form given on site. Narcotics Anonymous is a nonprofit, international, community-based organisation for recovering addicts.

The NSHN Forum (National Self-Harm Network)

www.nshn.co.uk

The National Self-Harm Network forum aims to support individuals who self harm to reduce emotional distress and improve their quality of life. They support and provide information for family and carers of individuals who self harm.

Patient UK

www.patient.co.uk

For general advice on health and medical conditions. Use the search box to find advice on depression and related conditions.

PsychNet-UK

www.psychnet-uk.com/

Tel: 0845 122 8622 (counselling line, 10.00am-1.00pm and 7.00pm-10.00pm, Monday to Friday)

A huge online source for medical information, including a section of mental health information and information on schizophrenia for professionals, families and students. Online support groups and links.

Rape Crisis England & Wales (Rape Crisis Federation)

www.rapecrisis.co.uk

Address: Suite E4, Josephs Well, Hanover Walk, Leeds LS3 1AB

Email: rcewinfo@rapecrisis.org.uk

Co-ordinates rape crisis centres around the country, and specialist services for women and girls who have experienced rape. Rape Crisis England & Wales (RCEW) is a feminist organisation that supports the work of Rape Crisis Centres across England and Wales. They work to raise awareness and understanding of sexual violence and abuse in all its forms.

Relate UK

www.relate.org.uk

Tel: Tel: 0300 1001234

This charity offers advice, relationship counselling, sex therapy, and has workshops, mediation consulting and face-to-face or phone counselling. To find your nearest Relate office telephone or use the inline email form.

Relationships Scotland

www.relationships-scotland.org.uk

Address: 18 York Place, Edinburgh, EH1 3EP

Tel: 0345 119 2020 (infoline)

Email: enquiries@relationships-scotland.org.uk

This Scottish charity was formed from the merger of Relate Scotland and Family Mediation Scotland. Relationships Scotland's network provides relationship counselling, family mediation, child contact centres and other family support services across all of mainland and island Scotland. Their work supports individuals, couples and families experiencing relationship difficulties.

SANE

www.sane.org.uk

Address: SANE, St. Mark's Studios, 14 Chillingworth Road, Islington, London N7 8QJ

Tel: 0300 304 7000 (helpline, open 4.30pm – 10.30pm daily) / 0203 805 1790 (office)

Email: info@sane.org.uk

SANE is a leading UK mental health charity.

UKNA (Narcotics Anonymous)

www.ukna.org

Address: 202 City Road, London, EC1V 2PH

Tel: 0300 999 1212 (helpline)

Email: meetings@ukna.org

This organisation is a voluntary community of people who have a drug problem and want to get help, regardless of what drug or combination of drugs have been used, and irrespective of age, sex, religion, race, creed or class. Narcotics Anonymous describes itself as a "non-profit fellowship or society of men and women for whom drugs have become a major problem". The group is made up of recovering addicts who meet regularly to help each other stay clean.

The UK National Work Stress Network

www.workstress.net

Address: 9 Bell Lane, Syresham, Brackley, NN13 5HP

Tel: Tel: 07966196033

Email: iandraper@nasuwt.net

Online tools, advice and guidance to help deal with stress in the workplace. Does not offer counselling but gives links to other organisations which do.

Verywell Health (About.com)

https://www.verywellhealth.com

Address: Dotdash, Inc., Attn: Verywell, 1500 Broadway, New York, NY 10036, USA

Tel: (US Number) 212-204-4000

Email: feedback@verywell.com

An American website with information on a range of conditions including depression in children and adults.

Your GP Surgery

Your local GP and practice nurse will be very happy to give you advice or point you in the direction of a local support group for any of the issues covered in this book.

Exercise Advice

The Keep Fit Association
www.keepfit.org.uk/
Tel: 01403 266000
Email: kfa@emdp.org
Brings people in similar areas together to exercise.

National Sports Agencies
These organisations are responsible for promoting sport and active lifestyles in their respective areas. They encourage people at all levels to get more involved in physical activity and are a good source of information if you are looking for advice about special activities and initiatives where you live.

Scotland: sportscotland
www.sportscotland.org.uk
Tel: 0141 534 6500
Email: sportscotland.enquiries@sportscotland.org.uk
Address: Doges, Templeton on the Green, 62 Templeton Street, Glasgow G40 1DA

England: Sport England
www.sportengland.org
Tel: 0345 8508 508
Email: funding@sportengland.org
Address: 21 Bloomsbury Street, London, WC1B 3HF

Wales: Sport Wales
http://sport.wales/
Tel: 0300 300 3111
Email: info@sportwales.org.uk
Address: Sport Wales, Sophia Gardens, Cardiff CF11 9SF

Northern Ireland: Sport NI
www.sportni.net
Tel: 028 9038 1222
Email: info@sportni.net
Address: 2a Upper Malone Road, Belfast BT9 5LA

Walking & Hiking Information
www.whi.org.uk
Email: contactus@whi.org.uk
A website with information about getting involved in walking and hiking, and ideas for places to go for the best walks.

Alternative Therapies

The Complementary and Natural Healthcare Council
www.cnhc.org.uk
Address: 83 Victoria Street, LONDON SW1H 0HW.
Tel: 0203 178 2199.
Email: info@cnhc.org.uk.
For information on complementary healthcare providers.

General Hypnotherapy Standards Council & General Hypnotherapy Register
www.general-hypnotherapy-register.com
Address: GHSC & GHR, PO BOX 204, Lymington S)41 6WP.
Email: admin@general-hypnotherapy-register.com
The General Hypnotherapy Standards Council (GHSC) and the General Hypnotherapy Register (GHR) are the UK's largest and most prominent organisations within the field of hypnotherapy and together present an exemplary model for the simultaneous protection of the public and the provision of practitioner credibility services.

Professional Organisations

BABCP – British Association for Behavioural and Cognitive Psychotherapies
www.babcp.com
Address: Imperial House, Hornby Street, Bury, Lancashire BL9 5BN
Tel: 0330 320 0851
Email: babcp@babcp.com
The BABCP is a multi-disciplinary interest group for people involved in the practice and theory of behavioural and cognitive psychotherapy. They aim to promote the development of the theory and practice of Behavioural and Cognitive Psychotherapies in all applicable settings in accordance with the Standards of Conduct Performance and Ethics.

British Association for Counselling and Psychotherapy

www.bacp.co.uk

Address: BACP House, 15 St John's Business Park, Lutterworth, Leicestershire, LE17 4HB

Tel: 01455 883300

Email: bacp@bacp.co.uk

The BACP work to help the general public, individuals and commissioners make better, more informed choices about the provision of counselling, and continue to raise the ethical and professional standards of the profession. Has helpdesk service to help clients find therapists. They promote and provide education and training for counsellors and psychotherapists working in either professional or voluntary settings.

Irish Association for Counselling and Psychotherapy

https://iacp.ie

Address: IACP, First Floor, Marina House, 11-13 Clarence Street, Dun Laoghaire, Co. Dublin

Tel: 00 353 1 2303536

Email: iacp@iacp.ie

IACP represent the interests of both client and Counsellor/Psychotherapist in Ireland.

Mayo Clinic

http://www.mayoclinic.org

Mayo Clinic is an American non-profit organisation committed to clinical practice, education and research, and providing expert, whole-person care to everyone who needs healing. There is an email form on site on the contacts page. Their mission is to inspire hope and contribute to health and wellbeing by providing the best care to every patient through integrated clinical practice, education and research.

Oxford Cognitive Therapy Centre

www.octc.co.uk

Address: Oxford Cognitive Therapy Centre, Warneford Hospital, Oxford, OX3 7JX

Tel: +44 (0)1865 902801

Email: octc@oxfordhealth.nhs.uk

This website gives information about a number of self-help and information booklets about cognitive behavioural therapy for depression, obsessive compulsive disorder, bulimia nervosa and anorexia nervosa, anxiety disorders and others. OCTC is a self-funding agency within Oxford Health NHS Trust which provides specialised cognitive behavioral therapy (CBT) services, particularly in teaching and training.

UKCP – UK Council for Psychotherapy

www.psychotherapy.org.uk

Address: 2 America Square, London EC3N 2LU

Tel: 020 7014 9955

Email: info@ukcp.org.uk

The UKCP are the leading organisation for the education, training, accreditation and regulation of psychotherapists and psychotherapeutic counsellors in the UK. They exist to promote and maintain high standards of practice of psychotherapy for the benefit of the UK public.

WHO – World Health Organisation

www.who.int/en/

Address: Avenue Appia 20, 1211 Geneva 27, Switzerland

Tel: + 41 22 791 21 11

Email: info@who.int

The primary role of the World Health Organisation is to direct and coordinate international health within the United Nations system.

Sources

House of Commons Defence Committee. *Mental Health and the Armed Forces, Part One: The Scale of mental health issues*, Eleventh Report of Session 2017–19.

How Common is PTSD in Veterans? - PTSD: National Center for PTSD
https://www.ptsd.va.gov/understand/common/common_veterans.asp

Journal of Abnormal Psychology. Vol 94(2), May 1985, 140-153: Life stressors and social resources affect post treatment outcomes among depressed patients. - Billings, Andrew G.; Moos, Rudolf H.

Maughan, Barbara et al. "Depression in childhood and adolescence." Journal of the Canadian Academy of Child and Adolescent Psychiatry = Journal de l'Academie canadienne de psychiatrie de l'enfant et de l'adolescent vol. 22,1 (2013): 35-40.

Mental health: 10 charts on the scale of the problem - BBC News
https://www.bbc.co.uk/news/health-41125009

Nearly a third of people are bullied at work, says TUC | TUC
https://www.tuc.org.uk/news/nearly-third-people-are-bullied-work-says-tuc

Seasonal affective disorder (SAD) - Symptoms and causes - Mayo Clinic
https://www.mayoclinic.org/diseases-conditions/seasonal-affective-disorder/symptoms-causes/syc-20364651